T0381793

THE CREATIVE TRANCE

In those moments when focus on creative work overrides input from the outside world, we are in a creative trance. This psychologically significant altered state of consciousness is inherent in everyone. It can take the form of daydreams generating scientific or creative ideas, hyperfocus in sports, visualizations that impact entire civilizations, life-changing audience experiences, or meditations for self-transformation that may access states beyond trance, becoming gateways to transcendence. Artist and psychologist Tobi Zausner shows how the creative trance not only operates in scientific inventions, sports, and works of art in all media but is also important in creating and recreating the self. Drawing on insights from cognitive neuroscience, clinical psychology, and post-materialist psychology, this book investigates the diversity of the creative trance ranging from nonindustrial societies to digital urban life, and its presence in people from all backgrounds and abilities. Finally, Zausner investigates the future of trance in our rapidly changing world.

TOBI ZAUSNER is a research psychologist, clinician, and award-winning visual artist. She is a Fellow of the American Psychological Association, a prolific presenter and writer, author of *When Walls Become Doorways: Creativity and the Transforming Illness* (2016), and has taught at the C. G. Jung Foundation, for Analytical Psychology, Saybrook University, Long Island University, and The New School.

THE CREATIVE TRANCE

Altered States of Consciousness and the Creative Process

TOBI ZAUSNER

C. G. Jung Foundation for Analytical Psychology, New York

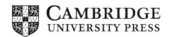

CAMBRIDGE
UNIVERSITY PRESS

University Printing House, Cambridge CB2 8BS, United Kingdom

One Liberty Plaza, 20th Floor, New York, NY 10006, USA

477 Williamstown Road, Port Melbourne, VIC 3207, Australia

314–321, 3rd Floor, Plot 3, Splendor Forum, Jasola District Centre,
New Delhi – 110025, India

103 Penang Road, #05–06/07, Visioncrest Commercial, Singapore 238467

Cambridge University Press is part of the University of Cambridge.

It furthers the University's mission by disseminating knowledge in the pursuit of
education, learning, and research at the highest international levels of excellence.

www.cambridge.org
Information on this title: www.cambridge.org/9781108488266
DOI: 10.1017/9781108769280

© Tobi Zausner 2022

First published 2022

A catalogue record for this publication is available from the British Library.

Library of Congress Cataloging-in-Publication Data
NAMES: Zausner, Tobi, author.
TITLE: The creative trance : altered states of consciousness and the creative process /
Tobi Zausner, PhD.
DESCRIPTION: 1 Edition. | New York, NY : Cambridge University Press, 2022. |
Includes bibliographical references and index.
IDENTIFIERS: LCCN 2021055083 (print) | LCCN 2021055084 (ebook) | ISBN 9781108488266
(hardback) | ISBN 9781108769280 (ebook)
SUBJECTS: LCSH: Altered states of consciousness. | Trance. | Creative ability. |
BISAC: PSYCHOLOGY / Applied Psychology
CLASSIFICATION: LCC BF1045.A48 Z38 2022 (print) | LCC BF1045.A48 (ebook) |
DDC 154.4–dc23/eng/20220113
LC record available at https://lccn.loc.gov/2021055083
LC ebook record available at https://lccn.loc.gov/2021055084

ISBN 978-1-108-48826-6 Hardback
ISBN 978-1-108-73858-3 Paperback

This book is dedicated to all daydreamers everywhere

Contents

Acknowledgments

It is my hope that this book will be an inspiration for the mind and the creativity of the reader. Many people have helped me on the journey to a completed manuscript, and I would like to thank them. Ruth Richards was there from the beginning with her wide academic expertise and pertinent suggestions. Stanley Krippner helped greatly with references to material that was esoteric yet quantified. Gloria Gaev offered perceptive structural recommendations, and Alan Leslie Combs gave enthusiastic support.

    I would like to thank the people at Cambridge University Press who helped bring this project to publication. First is the executive publisher, David Repetto, who had the courage to accept a work on post-materialist psychology. The content manager, Laura Simmons, carefully directed all the detailed production and scheduling, while the editorial assistants, Katie Idle, Emily Watton, and Harry James Morris, graciously made everything easier. I would also like to thank the many people that I cite in the book for their creativity and their willingness to make their creative process known.

The Pervasive State of Trance

Our normal waking consciousness, rational consciousness as we call it, is but one special type of consciousness, whilst all about it, parted from it by the filmiest of screens, there lie potential forms of consciousness entirely different

William James

Imagination is the landscape in which the artist goes for a walk

Meret Oppenheim

Trance as a Natural Pervasive State

Trance pervades our lives. Whenever we are creative, contemplative, or imaginative, lost in the world of a task, a daydream, or memories, we are in an altered state of consciousness, a state of trance. While some of these altered states are pure relaxation and others are dedicated solely to memory retrieval, there are states of trance that occur during creativity. In this book, the many altered states of the creative process are collectively called a *creative trance*. Inherent in every one of all backgrounds and abilities, the creative trance has transformed lives and changed the world. This psychologically significant altered state of consciousness reveals that our inner life is as important as our outer existence.

The Multiple Trance States of Creativity

The trance states essential to creativity can extend from the reveries of everyday life to transcendent experiences of universal unity. Fundamental to science, the arts, sports, spirituality, and recreating the self, the creative trance has revolutionized the course of civilizations. At age sixteen, Albert Einstein's (1879–1955) visualization of himself riding a light beam became a basis for his work in relativity theory (Weinstein, 2017). Elias Howe (1819–1867) discovered a key part to his invention of the sewing machine in a dream and the mathematician Srinivas Ramanujan (1887–1920) dreamt of his mathematical formulas (Harmon & Rheingold, 1984).

In a creative trance, the ego may willingly relinquish conscious control of the work. When Alice Walker (b. 1944) was writing her novel *The Color Purple*, she said its characters spoke with her and that "they were very obliging, engaging, and jolly" (cited in Currey, p. 118). The pianist Rosalyn Tureck (1913–2003) insists, "I do what Bach tells me to do. I never tell the music what to do" (cited in Mach, 1991, p. 169).

Immersion in a creative trance may be so complete that the outer world can seem to fade away. There may be no sense of discomfort, even during a time of extreme exertion. On running the mile in under four minutes, Roger Bannister (1929–2018) said he felt no pain and that the world appeared to stand still or not to exist; the only reality seemed to be the track beneath his feet (Bannister, 2018). The creative trance state may also appear like the entry into an auxiliary world. The cytogeneticist Barbara McClintock (1902–1992) imagined she was inside the corn cells she studied while viewing the mobility of their genetic elements (Keller, 1983), research that won her a Nobel Prize (Nobel Prize, 2021).

The creative trance can also be central to recreating the self. Jungian psychology uses active imagination, a type of guided meditation, to uncover the unconscious origins of emotional concerns. For Carl Jung (1875–1961), its founder, the inner life was both primary and spiritual. He said (Jung, 1963, p. 4), "In the end the only events in my life worth telling are those when the imperishable world erupted into this transitory one. That is why I speak chiefly of inner experiences, amongst which I include my dreams and visions."

The Creative Trance: Its Diversity and Antiquity

Creative trances are natural, varied, and widespread. The times of trance can last from the seconds of an epiphany or a flash of insight to the days and nights that the Tibetan meditative runners, the *lung-gom-pa*, took to cross the high plateau (David-Neel, 1971). Ranging from relaxation to rapture, states of trance are an essential aspect of human consciousness and distinct from waking awareness. Levels of a creative trance can vary from the light pleasant engagement in a task, congruent in many ways with Csikszentmihalyi's state of flow (1990, 1996), to a deeper absorption that seems to obliterate all sense of the external world. Occupying a greater part of life than is generally realized, they demonstrate that our daily perception of consensual reality is only one facet in the complexity of human consciousness.

The creative trance can also occur when we appreciate art, become lost in a story we are reading, or in a performance we are watching. Entering that state of receptive appreciation is entering an audience creative trance. These pervasive fluid states are a normal part of existence, and humans evolved to experience them. Evolutionary theorists find that we are built for creativity (Tooby & Cosmides, 2005), and suggest that altered states are an intrinsic capacity of the human nervous system (Lewis-Williams & Clottes, 1998). As a product of our evolution, creative trance states are an essential aspect of human culture.

The archaic origins of trance are intimated in Paleolithic artifacts suggesting the existence of altered states through initiation symbolism and the ritualized rebirth of the self. In North American Navajo sand paintings, a state leading to trance is induced through prayer to create space for the work (Krippner, 2008), and the Taoist painter Han Kan (c.718–780) felt that prayers inspired his brush (Sze, 1963). People of the Benin culture in Africa believe that the deity Olokun brings creativity in dreams and states of reverie (Krippner, 1999a), and Australian Aborigine artists depict their dreaming, which is in an altered state of Dreamtime, a parallel world of ancestors, spirits, and the divine (Caruana, 1993).

The Creative Trance: Disparagement and Inclusion

One of the most widespread aspects of the creative trance is also one of the most disparaged, and that is daydreaming. To an outside observer, the daydreamer may appear to accomplish nothing, but with certain individuals, these reveries can change the world. Einstein's visualizations were pivotal to his work in physics. Yet when he was a boy, Einstein's teacher told his parents that he was constantly "adrift" in his daydreams and "mentally slow" (Goertzel & Goertzel, 1962, p. 248). Thomas Alva Edison's (1847–1931) teacher called him "addled" and expelled him from school for daydreaming (Mould, 2016, p. 500), and Leonardo da Vinci (1452–1519) was reported to Ludovico Sforza, the Duke of Milan, for daydreaming instead of working (Vasari, 1996). Although often not apparent to the outside world, daydreams can be central to creativity.

The creative trance is not only diverse, occurring in individuals of all backgrounds, but is also inclusive with people of many different abilities experiencing altered states. Both disabilities and illness have the capacity to positively influence a creative trance. Different abilities may shape and augment the creative process, because they extend its parameters with the Paralympics, wheelchair dancing, and inclusive theatre and dance companies. As the world champion wheelchair dancer Piotr Iwanicki says, "When I'm on the dance floor, nothing matters at all. Dancing is all my life. It's my passion."

For some people, illness can reshape a creative trance and become the turning point to a new life and an experience of post-traumatic growth. I call this a *transforming illness* (Zausner, 2016). Itchiku Kubota (1917–2003) had a transforming illness by regarding his experience of acute hepatitis as "the time of deepest import in my life as an artist" (Kubota, 1984, p. 129). Afterward, he redesigned an ancient tradition of Japanese textiles and kimonos.

The Creative Trance: A Personal View

Inclusion is important to me because I have had both illness and disabilities. In 1989, I had a very aggressive type of ovarian cancer and even with an operation and chemotherapy, my doctors did not think I would survive. Yet after the illness my life changed. In addition to being a visual artist (which I still am), I also became a research psychologist. Years before that, I was inadvertently poisoned by an insecticide, but it was during the long recovery that my mature style of painting emerged.

For most of my life, until an operation in 2010 corrected my vision, I was legally blind without glasses. Although my extreme nearsightedness could be rectified with glasses and contact lenses, it still affected my creative trance because without them the world was a blur. My intense longing to see clearly expressed itself in my art, where all the images were painted or drawn with great clarity and not like the world that unassisted I could not see. I am also dyslexic and have attention-deficit hyperactivity disorder (ADHD). Without dyslexia, I would have been a physicist or mathematician, but often I cannot see all the numbers in an equation. I find that ADHD helps my creativity with its spurts of energy and its capacity for hyperfocus. Hyperfocus is excellent for a creative trance by strengthening concentration and intensifying the visualizations of possible trajectories for works in progress.

The research and title for this book, *The Creative Trance*, started over twenty years ago when I was studying the creativity of visual artists. In reading their biographies and writing, I became aware of the presence of many and varied altered states of consciousness in their creative processes.

In my personal experience as a visual artist, I have also experienced altered states of consciousness. Through extending this research into other disciplines, it became apparent that altered states shape the creative process across domains.

The Creative Trance as Acceptable and Valued

With their widespread occurrence, it is time to bring the altered states of a creative trance into the mainstream of creativity research and psychology research in general. As William James (1929) explained, we have multiple states of consciousness in addition to the waking awareness that was previously thought to completely dominate our lives. Now it appears that waking consciousness may share control with altered states during the creative process. Until this book, there has been no attempt to investigate the multiple aspects of a creative trance with its widespread cultural impact and occurrence across domains. By recognizing this altered state, we begin to acknowledge the vast and complex inner life that continually influences our existence, lays the foundation for consensual reality, and shapes human culture.

Through its emotional and cognitive resources, the creative trance can enhance personal growth and benefit society. By acknowledging this, we can create a more positive attitude toward our inner life and realize it is not an embarrassment but a source of inspiration. Destigmatizing the word and state of trance will generate increased scholarship in the field and provide greater access to creative potential. As a clinician I find the word *trance* makes some patients uncomfortable. Although they associate it with a fear of losing control, trance institutes a different kind of control, one that is aligned with exploration and awe.

Using the Word *Trance*

Yet, why use the word *trance* to describe these differing experiences of creative functioning? When this book was being reviewed, one of the reviewers likened its use of the word *trance* to Howard Gardner's (1985) use of the words *multiple intelligences* rather than *multiple talents* to describe the variety of human abilities. It was more controversial yet encouraged greater discussion. Calling a group of abilities an intelligence rather than a talent opened a world of possibilities and stimulated further investigation. It also gave people with abilities not previously considered to be an intelligence increased self-respect and may have encouraged them to further develop their capacities. It is possible that this investigation of the creative trance may have similar benefits.

What Gardner has done with multiple intelligences, this book purports to do with the extremely widespread and varied human capacity for trance. It is a word, a concept, and an ability that has been overlooked and pathologized. Yet it has enormous strength and comprises a greater part of life than is currently acknowledged. We are more than just our waking cognition. Noncognitive processes, such as emotions, feelings, intuitions, and perceptions, are wide ranging and many of them are also related to trance states. Revealing their connection to each other and to the creative trance will allow them to be understood and appreciated with new insight. This process can bring previously hidden aspects of the mind into the open for further discourse and study.

The specific term *creative trance* appears to be unique to this research and is intended to introduce a new concept to scholarship and life. Identifying trance as a natural state of consciousness with a connection to creativity makes it more available and acceptable to personal experience. Just as the unconscious plays a greater role in our life than is generally acknowledged (Bargh, 2005; Wegner, 2005), so do instances of trance shape our ongoing existence. In a creative trance, we can access more information than is usually available to our conscious mind and by bringing this information into conscious awareness, the creative trance becomes a goal-achieving inner journey, a vacation with purpose.

Negative Inner States

Of course, not all interior states are positive instances of a creative trance. Some may be symptoms of dissociative disorders (APA, 2020) or an immobilization in response to trauma. Negative states may also mirror adverse facets of emotional life and express themselves as rumination, obsession, or perseveration (World Health Organization, 1992; American Psychiatric Association, 2013). Yet, in the clinical aspects of a creative trance, analyzing what appears to be an obstruction may become a key to individuation.

The Chapters of the Creative Trance

Chapter One: The Multifaceted Creative Trance: In those moments, or seconds, or hours, when focus on our creative work overrides input from the outside world, we are in the altered state of a creative trance. Shaped by individual experiences, social circumstances, and cultural traditions, the creative trance is multifaceted and psychologically significant, taking numerous forms throughout the sciences, the arts, sports, and in audience responsiveness. For Lynn Margulis, inspiration from nature was a creative trance, observations that led to her theory of symbiogenesis, the importance of symbiosis in evolution. The multiple depths of a creative trance, from light flow states to a deep immersion that obliterates all external stimuli, possibly correlate with the psychological capacity for absorption. The audience creative trance of reception can extend from enjoyment to the overwhelming Stendhal syndrome.

Chapter Two: Consciousness and Creativity Theory in the Creative Trance: Creativity, an apex of consciousness, contains the altered states of a creative trance. Ranging from quiet reveries to fast-moving sports, the creative trance can also be a transcendent experience, an ecstasy using the body's own pharmacology. It can be the inner focus of both Mozart and Shostakovich, who composed finished music in their minds. The creative trance relates to the five factor model of personality, openness, Big-C and little-c creativity, Wallas' four-stage creative process, and Barron's concept of a habitually creative person. Cross-culturally, meditation and sleep are central to a creative trance. The Native North American Chippewa weave dream images into their beadwork and banners; in India, the Saroa decorate the walls of their homes with images from their dreams.

Chapter Three: Unconscious Origins of the Creative Trance: We live in a multiplicity of personal worlds, all connected through the power of our unconscious mind and its capacity for trance. Unlike the slow sequential conscious mind, the larger unconscious is a parallel processor, combining multiple variables to bring depth and complexity into the creative process. Relinquishing conscious creative control can become an artistic projective identification. As the visual artist Joan Mitchell says, "The painting tells me what to do." The cognitive unconscious, with its perceptual-cognitive abilities, automated motor skills, and implicit memory, facilitates creative expression while our unconscious emotions, internal conflicts, and repressed desires drive the inspiration and passion of a creative trance. Unconscious automatic actions can generate fluid expertise, as in the violinist no longer concentrating on finger positions and the archer instinctually positioning a bow.

Chapter Four: Empathy and Dissociation in the Creative Trance: Empathy and dissociation, seemingly opposites, form a paradoxical union in the creative trance. Inherently structured by domain, cultural traditions, personal preferences, and rules to achieve excellence, the creative trance is empathic, connecting the creative person with the work produced, and dissociative, separating trance states from waking consciousness. Athletes use empathy to intuit the moves of an opponent. In science, the inventor Alexander Graham Bell felt he became one with his machines; and Stanislavski's system of empathic acting revolutionized film and theater. Some empathic people view creative products as their children, while dissociative inspiration can seem to originate from a muse or divine source. Dissociation in ritual trance possession with dancers assuming the identity of deities may bring numinous experiences for both performers and audience.

Chapter Five: Evolution, Altered States, and the Creative Trance: We are creative primates who evolved from creative primates and as our cognition increased, so did the complexity of our creative trance. In the evolutionary history of our symbolic communication, even early works suggest altered states and transformation of the self. There are archaic artifacts with symbols that intimate initiation and life after death, prehistoric images on cave walls intended to influence both affect and reality, and talismanic objects linked to altered states, rituals, pain relief, and healing. Beginning with everyday needs, our creativity advanced from simple Lomekwian and Oldowan stone tools to Paleolithic ritual objects with archetypal symbolism encoding spiritual rebirth, to plans that could alter civilizations, expanding human cognitive capacity with external memory devices like alphabets, computers, and the digital cloud.

Chapter Six: The Creative Trance and the Brain: The mind is the seat of trance. Every thought we have, every movement we make, changes the landscape of our brain and our creative trance. Every thought produces its own neural signature, from insights into everyday problems to the meditative neuroplasticity of transcendent states. With its unique assembly of neural processes, creativity is associated with the release of dopamine, endorphins, serotonin, and oxytocin, and can be shaped by insight and synesthesia. Cognitive neuroscience reveals the heterogeneity of creative trance states through activation of different brain regions, such as the medial temporal lobe memory network, the prefrontal cortex, both brain hemispheres, and significantly the default mode network, which is associated with divergent thinking and daydreaming. As the Nobel Prize winning pharmacologist James Black said, "I daydream like mad."

Chapter Seven: Dynamics of the Creative Trance: We live an unpredictable unrepeatable yet creative existence. Revealing the underlying patterns of our thoughts and behavior, nonlinear dynamics provides models to understand our lives and creativity as ever-evolving human beings in a constantly changing universe. The creative trance, modeled as a creative chaos, brings forth new work and personal transformation. With its disciplines of chaos theory and complexity theory, nonlinear dynamics explains processes like creativity that do not progress in a straight line, are not predictable, never exactly repeat themselves, and yet have the capacity for originality and transformation. Aspects of nonlinear dynamics such as attractors, fractals, self-organization, emergence, sensitivity to initial conditions, also known as the butterfly effect, and self-organized criticalities strongly correlate with the creative process, insights, the power of memories, global transformation, catharsis, and transforming panic attacks into creativity.

Chapter Eight: Dyslexia, Attention-Deficit Disorder, and the Creative Trance: Whatever affects the brain structures the creative trance, and what we view as imperfections may instead be alternate pathways to achievement. No one is perfect but as Jung says, we have an inner dynamic wholeness that transcends perfection and fuels self-evolution. The creative people in this chapter use dyslexia and attention-deficit disorder, now known as attention-deficit hyperactivity disorder (ADHD), to access their wholeness, and this in turn drives and shapes their creative trance. Eminent writers with dyslexia include Agatha Christie, William Butler Yeats, Jules Verne, and F. Scott Fitzgerald. Frank Lloyd Wright used the reveries of ADHD to create completed works of architecture in his mind; and Leonardo da Vinci, who had both dyslexia and ADHD, changed the course of Western art history.

Chapter Nine: Illness and Transformation in the Creative Trance: Just as illness and difficulties punctuate our lives, so do times of healing and achievement. As an experience of recovery and renewal, healing through self-expression is a creative process and a triumph of the creative trance, bringing a new self and new work. Addressing both emotional and physical pain, healing can occur in the creative arts therapies or individually. Using her creativity in a hope to heal the world, Greta Thunberg also healed her speaking difficulties. Paradoxically, impairments may augment the creative trance by becoming a transforming illness, as in Ludwig van Beethoven's increasing deafness that imparted greater power to his music. Even when a condition is terminal and there is no cure, healing can occur with an altered yet profound form of creative trance.

Chapter Ten: Different Abilities and the Creative Trance: Different abilities enlarge the terrain of the creative trance by demonstrating the extended capacities of human beings. Challenges widen the possibilities for everyone. Not all conditions can be "cured," but healing is always available through self-transformation. Differently abled people experience altered states in sports competitions, the Paralympics, dance, wheelchair dance, music, writing, performances, science, and visual art, sometimes without limbs, vision, or hearing. They share a triumph of achievement gained through accomplishing something that was once thought to be impossible – perhaps even by them. There are now physically integrated dance and theater companies for people of all abilities and a long lineage of blind African American music professionals. The effort to confront impediments alters the neural landscapes of their brains and empowers their creative trance.

Chapter Eleven: Dementia and the Creative Trance: Worldwide, we are an aging population with dementia affecting people in increasing numbers. Here we focus on two types of dementia: Alzheimer's disease, the most prevalent form of dementia, and the primary progressive aphasia of fronto-temporal dementia because of its capacity to enhance creativity in music and visual art. For individuals with dementia, the creative trance can be an oasis apart from their daily world of growing difficulties. Instead, they face the solvable problems of creativity. Iris Murdoch wrote her final novel, *Jackson's Dilemma*, during the early stages of Alzheimer's disease, and Willem de Kooning focused on painting as his dementia advanced. Sometimes, dementia can influence work for the better even if only for a brief time. Frontotemporal dementia gave power to Maurice Ravel's best-known music *Bolero*.

Chapter Twelve: Altered States of a Lifesaving Creative Trance: Creative trance states can extend to lifesaving acts of heroism that far exceed ordinary human limitations. By entering a creative trance in the middle of a raging forest fire, the firefighter Wag Dodge discovered a new way to reroute the path of flames. Altered states may also occur when individuals lift a multi-thousand-pound vehicle to rescue a person trapped beneath it. They display what is colloquially called *hysterical strength*, which this book calls *extraordinary human strength* (EHS). In EHS, there is a possible dominance of the dorsal system of the brain with the potential effects of adrenaline, norepinephrine, and cortisol, and correspondences to the yoga philosophy of Patanjali. The enormous power of EHS may derive from quantum sources and neural quantum processes, with correlates in Eastern philosophies.

Ranging from solutions to everyday problems, to insights that construct new pathways in science and the arts, to feats of heroism that appear to extend the laws of physics and the physiological capacities of human beings, the creative trance is simultaneously central to life and the great power that drives the edges of achievement forward.

CHAPTER I

The Multifaceted Creative Trance

Great creativity is responsible for humanity's great achievements
Silvano Arieti

The brain is wider than the sky
Emily Dickinson

In those moments, or seconds, or hours, when focus on our creative work overrides input from the outside world, we are in the altered state of a creative trance. Like a multifaceted diamond, with each facet shining, each illuminating the others leading back to its core, the creative trance has multiple aspects driven by the core of our unconscious mind. There are as many instances of the creative trance as there are creative people and occurrences of their creativity. Shaped by individual experiences, environmental circumstances, differing physical capacities, and diverse cultural traditions, the creative trance takes numerous forms.

Appearing differently in everyone, the creative trance is ubiquitous, identifiable, yet always unique. A metaphor for its multiple manifestations and individual aspects would be William Blake's description of sunshine, "the suns light when he unfolds it, depends on the organ that beholds it" (Blake, 1820, Frontispiece). The phenomenology of the creative trance is vast, appearing in the sciences, the arts, clinical modalities, sports, self-transformation, and the pursuit of well-being. In its spiritual forms, the creative trance can become a gateway to states beyond trance, intimations of the ineffable and universal oneness. Yet each trance originates in the private world of a creative person.

Multiple Aspects of the Creative Trance

Our mental lives manifest as a stream of thought (James, 1918), phenomenal reality presenting "itself as a changing display of experience" (Combs

& Krippner, 2003, p. 48). Within our ongoing stream of awareness are altered states of consciousness that this book collectively calls a *creative trance*. They can occur whenever we are creative, imaginative, or contemplative, lost in the world of a daydream or memories, or engaged in a task. These altered states may intensify when we are immersed in an inner world so deeply that the interior space feels like our primary reality. Then bodily discomforts may vanish even during prolonged exertion, although we continue to remain in the physical world. The physician and athlete Roger Bannister (1929–2018) described this experience when running to break the barrier of the four-minute mile. "There was no pain, only a great unity of movement and aim. The world seemed to stand still or did not exist. The only reality was the next two hundred yards of track under my feet" (Bannister 2018, p. 171).

Contents of the trance state can vary widely from the relaxation of daydreaming to envisioning plans that impact entire civilizations. Distinct from the entropic trance states of catatonia, stupor, daze, and addiction, the creative trance can improve health and in certain cases can alter the world. The physicist Albert Einstein's (1879–1955) visualization of himself at age sixteen riding a light beam later became a basis for his theory of special relativity that transformed physics (Weinstein, 2017). The machinist turned inventor Elias Howe (1819–1867) dreamt the solution to his invention of the sewing machine (Harmon & Rheingold, 1984), a discovery that revolutionized the textile industry, creating mass-produced clothing and employment opportunities for women.

The biologist and evolutionary theorist Lynn Margulis (1938–2011) took her inspiration from nature (Feldman, 2018). What another person might see as only scum on a pond or puddle was for Margulis an experience of delight, a creative trance. These observations of nature eventually led to her theory of symbiogenesis, the importance of symbiosis in evolution. Sometimes a creative trance can feel like the entry into an alternative world. When the cytogeneticist Barbara McClintock (1902–1992) was studying the genetics of corn, she felt she was inside the corn cell along with its chromosomes (Keller, 1983). Through her research, McClintock discovered the mobility of genetic elements and won the 1983 Nobel Prize in Physiology or Medicine (Nobel Prize, 2021).

Creativity and the Creative Trance

Creativity requires the capacity to receive stimuli from our external and internal worlds, the ability to connect these disparate pieces of information through conscious and unconscious processing, and the necessary work that brings the creative products into consensual reality. All these steps are aspects of a creative trance. Creativity, as the driving center of the creative trance, permeates our existence, ranging from the everyday creativity of daily life, such as cooking, gardening, building bookcases, and problem-solving (Richards, 2007), to the peak of eminent creativity with art and science that define a civilization.

The two criteria generally associated with creativity are originality and usefulness (Richards, 2018), but Barron (1969, p. 20) believes there should be an additional property of "elegance" or "aesthetic fit." He also notes that because human beings cannot create something from nothing, all human creativity is the reorganization of existing materials, and that distinguished creative achievement almost invariably takes hard work, dedication, and continued practice.

Definitions of Trance

Although there are many definitions of *trance*, for the purposes of this book, I will use one of the definitions from the *American Psychological Association Dictionary of Psychology*, which defines *trance* as "an altered state of consciousness characterized by decreased awareness of and responsiveness to stimuli and an apparent loss of voluntary power" (APA, 2020, online). According to the American Psychological Association (APA), trance is an altered state of consciousness very different from the experience of ordinary wakefulness and may be accompanied by increased suggestibility and a reduction in voluntary power. The APA associates trance with hypnosis and delineates three levels of hypnotic trance: light, medium, and deep, defining all three levels as altered states of consciousness. Hypnosis may be induced either by a hypnotist or by autosuggestion. We will see that the creative trance also has varying layers of depth and, like the hypnotic trance, they may be facilitated by the capacity for absorption. The evolutionary theorists David Lewis-Williams and Jean Clottes (1998, pp. 14–15) believe that trance states "are wired into the human nervous system."

Current research extends the definition of trance to include its occurrence in states of meditation, relaxation, creativity, dissociation, shamanism, mediumship, and parapsychological phenomena (Krippner, 2002; Krippner & Combs, 2002; Hageman et al., 2010). I believe that all these states, as well as dreaming, the hypnagogic state just before sleep, and the hypnopompic state between sleep and waking, contain the capacity to become a creative trance. Additionally, the creative trance may be described as a purposeful altered state of consciousness focusing on creative work and bringing that work back into consensual reality. Kapchan (2007) finds trance to be a transcultural phenomenon that manifests in a cultural framework, and Grosso (1997, p. 193), who notes that creativity is a dissociative experience, calls it a "creative dissociation."

Tooby and Cosmides (2010, p. 176) say that "humans have evolved specialized cognitive machinery that allows us to enter and participate in imagined worlds." While they do not use the word *trance*, they describe this state as a *cognitive decoupling*. Madhill (1999), Gowan (1975), and Ghiselin (1952) connect creativity with a trance state. Madhill identifies what Richards (2018) calls everyday creativity as an everyday trance, describing it as an often-used adaptive mechanism to enhance impulse control and encourage a focus on work. While Ghiselin believes that the trance state of creativity is never directly induced but generated as part of the creative process, there appear to be multiple instances of trance induction before creative activity.

Trance Induction before Creativity

Cross-culturally, there are a variety of states preceding trance that facilitate creativity. In religious or spiritual settings, such as Tibetan and Navajo sand paintings (Krippner, 2008; Davis, 2016), a state leading to trance is induced through prayers to create space for the work. In China, Taoist and Buddhist artists have historically engaged in prayer and meditation to manifest a creative trance before beginning their work (Sze, 1963). The Taoist painter Han Kan (c. 718–780) believed that his brush became inspired because of his prayers. It was thought that preparing to paint is like preparing to meet an honored guest. In the Western tradition, the writer Alice Walker (b. 1944) said, "In order to invite any kind of guest, including creativity, you have to make room for it" (cited in Currey, 2019, p. 118). To facilitate a creative trance state, the poet Friedrich Schiller (1759–1895) liked to smell rotten apples, which he kept inside his desk, and the poet Wystan Hugh Auden (1907–1973) drank multiple cups of tea (Spender, 1985).

The bathtub, perhaps because of its relaxing womb-like quality of immersion in water, has long been used to inspire a creative trance (M. H., 2019). Perhaps its most famous incident of inspiration is the story of Archimedes (288 BCE–212 BCE), who rose out of his bath shouting *Eureka!* after discovering the measurement of volume and laws of buoyancy. The writers Franz Kafka (1883–1924) and Douglas Adams (1952–2001) and the visual artist Salvador Dali (1904–1989) all found that taking baths generated creative ideas. Winston

Churchill (1874–1965) used baths to inspire his strategic thinking, and the composer Benjamin Britten (1913–1976) required two baths per day, a very cold one in the morning and a very hot bath at night.

Trance states can also manifest when creative people arrange their materials in preparation for work. It becomes a secular ritual of the creative process. I remember my first formal oil painting lessons at age nine and the instructions for setting up a palette. The paints had to be in a specific color order, with the warm to cool tones across the top of the palette and the earth tones down the side. Once this order had been established, a sense of rightness emerged, and I could feel an internal shift. It was as if the door to a universe had opened, and I became ready to paint.

Dreaming the Creative Trance: Its Manifestation in Sleep and Associated States

It is also possible to use dream incubation as an induction with sleep as the trance state. Dream incubation is a process of directing the mind before sleep to solve a problem while dreaming and remember the solution when awake. Dream incubation, which was a common practice in ancient Egypt, China, Tibet, and Greece, was also used by the native tribes of the North American Plains (Krippner, 1999b). Across cultures and throughout time, sleep and its associated states have been venues for the creative trance. Barrett (2010, p. x) calls the prevalence of inspiration in sleep states "a different mode of thought – that supplements and enriches what we have already done while awake." Even when creative solutions appear in a similar form, such as a dream or the hypnagogic state before sleep, or the hypnopompic state before waking, the creative trance is always specific to the person who experiences it.

Dreams have been pivotal to the creative process. The writer John Steinbeck (1902–1968) believed that problems with creativity could be resolved by the "committee of sleep," and the poet St. Paul Roux (1861–1940) would hang a sign on the door of his bedroom stating, "Poet at work" (Barrett, 2010, p. ix). The machinist turned inventor Elias Howe (1819–1867) dreamt the solution to his sewing machine, and the mathematician Srinivas Ramanujan (1887–1920) dreamt of mathematical formulas (Harmon & Rheingold, 1984). In music, the composer Ludwig van Beethoven (1770–1827) dreamt an 1821 composition while napping in a carriage (Krippner, 1999a), and in visual art, Al Hirschfeld (1903–2003) dreamt his solutions to the drawings he made for the theater section of the *New York Times* (Currey, 2014).

A creative trance can also manifest in the half-awake times before and after sleep. The chemist Friedrich August Kekulé von Stradonitz (1829–1896) saw his discovery of the structure of the benzene molecule in a hypnagogic state, and the composer Richard Wagner (1813–1883) found the inspiration for the first opera of his *Ring Cycle* in a hypnagogic state (Krippner, 1999a). The writer Mary Shelley (1797–1851) conceived the idea for her novel *Frankenstein* (Shelley, 1831/1994) while in a hypnagogic state, and the inventor Thomas Edison (1847–1931) found that creative ideas filled his mind during his half-waking states (Krippner, 1999a). For the contralto Marian Anderson (1897–1993), the time before sleep was when she lived in the "mood of the music . . . lost in the spirit of the song," and said, "while all is still around one, a great deal is accomplished" (cited in Currey, 2019, p. 88).

Inspirational dreams and associated altered states are acknowledged across cultures. People of the Benin culture in Africa believed that the deity Olokun inspired creativity through dreams and states of reverie (Krippner, 1999a). For Australian Aborigines, Dreamtime is a place of both dreams and meditative states, a parallel world of ancestors, spirits, and the divine (Caruana, 1993). In paintings, they depict their Dreaming, an altered state of Dreamtime and a major inspiration for their art. In North America, the Chippewa weave dream images into their beadwork and banners; in India, the Saroa decorate the walls of their homes with images from their dreams (Barrett, 2010).

The Creative Trance: Its Contents, Time Frames, and Paradox

Creativity is inherent in human nature (Richards, 2007), and because of this, we all have the possibility of entering a creative trance. It can happen in our lives during times of focus on a project, or through relaxation, or in any instance when the unconscious mind generates an expanded awareness. While daydreaming, sleep dreaming, meditation, visualizations, and deep engagement in the creative process are easily associated with altered states of consciousness, even waking life has its multiple moments of trance. These instances might be of such short duration, lasting only moments or even seconds, that they may be considered micro trances. Brief trances in waking life could be the intuitive flashes of insight that bring clarity to help resolve everyday problems or fleeting but vivid memories of the past brought forth by a seemingly unimportant stimulus in the present.

They can also be of longer duration, such as an intuitive response or "hunch" about a person or situation, or any time that we are on autopilot, performing actions without our full focus or awareness. The time frames of a trance state may further increase to the extended meditations of the *lung-gom-pa* monks, who ran for days in an altered state across the Tibetan Plateau (David-Neel, 1971).

As a paradoxical fusion of opposites, the creative trance is a crucible that creates the new. It is a state of active passivity that is simultaneously dissociative yet operational. The creative trance is also internally focused, yet outwardly directed and highly functional. While psychologically experiencing what appears to be part of a personal or ultimate reality, creative individuals are also able to operate in the consensual or baseline reality. It is this fusion that creates the new work of art and the new self.

Multiple Facets of the Creative Trance: Its Variation across and within Domains

A creative trance can range from the quiet enjoyment of a relaxing creative activity, such as reading or needlepoint, that is a treasured but circum-scribed time in daily life to an altered state of consciousness extending throughout the creative process of a major work. Both Johannes Brahms (1833–1897) and Giacomo Puccini (1858–1924) spoke about being in an altered state while composing their music, and Johann Wolfgang von Goethe (1749–1832) said he was in a trance when writing his novel *Werther* (Harmon & Rheingold, 1984). It can be a feeling of creative possession where an idea takes hold and will not let go until it is expressed in physical form. The creative trance can also be the joy of movement in the present moment or a stillness and silence that feels like a transcendent experience outside of time.

Even within a creative domain, there are great differences. For some visual artists, painting is an agitated activity, while others appear to be calm. The Taoist dragon painter Ch'en Jung (c. 1200–1266), known for his "tempestuous nature," would sometimes paint "in a wild and furious manner splashing the ink and spitting in the water" (Sickman & Soper, 1956, p. 268). Louis Bouché (1896–1969) said, "I get very excited when I paint. My blood pressure goes up like the devil" (cited in Eliot, 1957, p. 210). In contrast, the surrealist artist René Magritte (1898–1967) worked meticulously. He painted quietly at an easel set up near a window in the corner of his living room that was filled with upholstered furniture and an Oriental rug (Gablik, 1970).

The creative trance also varies in sports performance. It may be an extreme hyperfocus on the present moment, with pinpoint mindfulness guiding precision movements. This was the experience of the world surfing champion Bernard "Midget" Farrelly (1955–2016), whose most creative times came when control, balance, and coordination combined to inspire daring and original movements on the surfboard (Murphy & White, 1995). Or it can be the runner Roger Bannister's deep trance state when the world appeared to stand still or be nonexistent (Bannister, 2018/1955).

Multiple Facets of the Creative Trance: Reveries, Planning, and Metaphysical States

Otherworldly experiences can also be part of the creative trance in visual art. Australian Aborigines have metaphysical experiences when they visit the Dreamtime, the world of their spirits (Caruana, 1993), and prehistoric cave paintings are now considered to be products of religious states that aim to convey an otherworldly response in the viewer (Clottes & Lewis-Williams, 1998).

Leonardo da Vinci (1452–1519) found the creative trance necessary for visual art and for scientific invention (Zausner, 2016). Although aggravating his patrons by what they considered to be excessive daydreaming and not working, Leonardo used his reveries to visualize his paintings and to invent machines, such as a helicopter, a bicycle, a parachute, an underwater breathing device, and a human-powered glider (da Vinci, 1970a,b). When accused of inactivity, Leonardo defended himself. He said that sometimes people accomplish more when they appear not to be working because the mind is then most active, and the mind must first imagine what the hands will later create (Vasari, 1996). The inventor Nikola Tesla (1856–1943) also visualized machines in his creative process (Cheney, 1981; Martin, 1992). Tesla would start the machines working in his mind and then check on them later to see if they needed adjustments.

For most people, the creative trance is both a mental state of planning and a physical state of making the work, but for some individuals, the mental state is where they do a major part of their creativity. Both Wolfgang Amadeus Mozart (1756–1791) (Holmes, 1845/2013) and Dmitry Shostakovich (1906–1975) (Currey, 2014) composed finished music in their heads before writing it down with few corrections. Alice Walker (b. 1944) says she needs a gestation time of one to two years of concentrated thinking about a novel before she writes anything (Currey, 2019). Yet when Walker begins writing, she writes very quickly.

Horace Pippin (1888–1946) visualized every detail of his paintings before he picked up a brush to create them. Pippin said that his paintings came to him, explaining, "I do over the picture several times in my mind and when I am ready to paint, I have all the details I need" (cited in Bearden, 1976, n.p.). The architect Frank Lloyd Wright (1867–1959) visualized his buildings so completely that he made very few preparatory sketches before presenting the final design to a client (Currey, 2014). Wright's capacity for intensive visualization appears to derive from his early life. When Wright was a child, his states of trancelike daydreaming were so deep that his uncle had to shout at the boy to return him to waking reality (Cramond, 1994).

Sports, theater, dance, and the pursuit of well-being all utilize states of trance and have a history of trance with roots in antiquity. There are the masked dramas of ancient Greece, the meditative trance runners of Japan, the ritual temple dancers of Southeast Asia, the ancient lineages of tribal dance in Africa and the Americas, and the healing systems of yoga and Qigong. These disciplines also address the spiritual aspect of life with its focus on the extended nonmaterial self. This concept, now researched in the domain of post-materialist psychology, includes pharmacologically assisted trance states to evoke changes in consciousness for the terminally ill.

The Audience Creative Trance: Receptive and Unique

For every work of art, there is both a trance of creation and a trance of reception, what this book calls an *audience creative trance*. The singer Nina Simone (1933–2003) said that she consciously created a trance state in her audience by directing their mood through her choice of songs and the order in which she presented them (Simone & Cleary, 2003). Yet anytime we are "carried away" by music, or whenever we enter the world of a book we are reading or a film we are watching, and the reality of the narrative overrides our sense of self-awareness, we are in an audience creative trance.

This active surrender (Winterson, 1997) in an audience trance is a creative response because it is unique to every individual. Generated by personal experience and preferences leading to the circumstances surrounding the moment of reception, no two people will have the same reaction. The individual response of each trance experience is fundamental to its use in healing modalities. It is central in the creative arts therapies and in clinical work, where altered states promote individuation through hypnosis, dream analysis, Jungian active imagination, EMDR (eye movement desensitization and reprocessing), and energy psychology.

The Quantified Audience Creative Trance: Resonance, Entrainment, and Synchronization

When we experience appreciation in an audience creative trance, we might resonate with and be entrained by the entertainment, unconsciously synchronizing our physiology with other spectators and with the performers. Synchronized behavior is prevalent throughout our universe, where fireflies, pendulums, electrons, and the pacemaker cells in a heart can all synchronize their actions (Strogatz, 2003). The emergence of synchronization in an audience creative trance may be an example of interaction adaptation theory, where behavior rather than cognitive planning generates mutually influencing exchanges (Burgoon & White, 2013). The degrees of synchronization and entrainment function as levels of resonance, which this book would identify as the different depths of an audience creative trance.

These states, distinctly separate from ordinary waking awareness, can be measured in quantified studies. By monitoring heartbeats and electrodermal responses in twelve audience attendees at a live musical theater performance in London's West End, researchers at University College London and Lancaster University found that their hearts were beating in unison (UCL, 2017). They also found that the audience members' pulse rates were increasing and decreasing in synchrony whether they knew each other or not. According to the lead psychologist Joe Devlin, "Experiencing the live theatre performance was extraordinary enough to overcome group differences and produce a common physiological experience in the audience members" (UCL, 2017, n.p.).

The Quantified Audience Creative Trance: Resonance and Synchronization with Performers

We may also have an audience creative trance through resonance with the performers, and in certain instances, live performances may elicit a greater response than taped events. Using transcranial magnetic stimulation, Jola and Grosbras (2013) measured stronger spectator reactions to live solo performances of ballet, the Indian dance of Bharatanatyam, and acting than to video recordings. They suggest that the spectators' increased motor corticospinal activity while observing the live performers indicates physical resonance and a possible activation of the mirror neuron system. This response may additionally imply kinesthetic empathy.

Two studies of spectator response during live modern dance concerts choreographed by Myriam Gourfink (b. 1968) also found audience entrainment, resonance, and evidence of mirror neuron activation (Bachrach et al., 2015; Joufflineau et al., 2018). Cardiovascular and respiratory measurements revealed physiological entrainment, while questionnaires evaluated cognitive entrainment though quantified measures of time distortion. Based on yoga and breathing techniques of meditation, Gourfink's choreography (Gourfink, 2005) is hypnotically slow and performed with attention to breath in a trancelike state of consciousness. Through kinesthetic resonance, some spectators appeared to enter an altered state like that of the dancers, which Bachrach and associates (2015, p. 12) call a "sharing of body-mind states." Yoga philosophy (Patanjali, 2011) addresses this extended consciousness by noting that breathing and concentration can bring deep synchrony and formless integration with the object of focus.

Collective Effervescence and the Audience/Participant Communal Creative Trance

There are creative trances that blur the line between audience and participant, with many people in both roles. This can happen at events with significant audience participation, such as festivals and weddings where people may dance as well as listen to music. By producing contagious energy, festive events may generate spontaneous organized behaviors, such as clapping, singing, and dancing. Exuberant circle dances that manifest this energy can also increase it with the joy of positive participation. Group dancing may provide access to the altered states of extending beyond one's personal boundaries to be part of a larger whole. The Italian tarantella, the Balkan and Jewish hora, the Kalamatianos of Greece, and the sardana of Spanish Catalonia are among its many examples.

This very active engaged altered state of communal audience/participant creative trance is what sociologist Émile Durkheim (1858–1917) calls *collective effervescence* (Durkheim, 1915, p. 219). Deriving from his work with Australian tribal populations, including the Warrunga, the Uluuru, and the Kingilli, Durkheim observed that their religious ceremonies created a type of communal rapture with sentiments shared from mind to mind that became expressed through song and dance. He observed that (p. 219) "a sort of electricity is formed" when people come together, and that it "transports them to an extraordinary degree of exaltation." Durkheim believed that collective effervescence could engender an experience of being beyond oneself that may lead to a spiritual awakening with intimations of the sacred and divine.

The Audience Creative Trance: The Stendhal Syndrome

One of the most dramatic incidences of an individual audience creative trance is the Stendhal syndrome. Identified by Graziella Magherini (1989), who was head of psychiatry at Santa Maria Nuova Hospital in Florence, it is a tourist's overwhelming psychological and sometimes also physical response to a work of art. Magherini named the response after the French author Stendhal (born Marie-Henri Beyle, 1783–1842), who wrote about having this type of extreme reaction in 1817 while traveling in Italy. Stendhal was psychologically and physically overcome by the beautiful frescoes and paintings of the Santa Croce chapel in Florence (Palacios-Sánchez et al., 2018). The chapel also contained the tombs of Galileo, Machiavelli, and Michelangelo. While experiencing what he said was a sublime ecstasy in response to the art, Stendhal also had a highly irregular heartbeat and extreme muscle weakness in his legs, to the extent that he feared he might fall.

Magherini (1989) observed over one hundred cases of tourists having extreme reactions to art. With symptoms ranging from anxiety and panic attacks to transient psychoses, she viewed them as previously repressed psychological problems manifesting in response to art and called them the Stendhal syndrome (Griffiths, 2014). The neurosurgeon Edson Amâncio (2005) believes that the writer Fyodor Dostoevsky (1821–1881) showed aspects of the Stendhal syndrome when he saw a painting of the *Dead Christ*, 1521–1522, by Hans Holbein the Younger (1497–1543) in the Basel Museum. Two years after visiting the museum, Dostoevsky published his novel, *The Idiot*, where the main character, Hippolite, also experiences an extreme reaction to the Holbein painting (Garcia-Fenech, 2019).

The Audience Creative Trance: Sacred and Healing

The healing response is fundamental to sacred ceremonies that create an audience trance of participation, such as the Navajo sandpaintings of Native North America (Reichard, 1977). These paintings, made of naturally pigmented dry sands and constructed while chanting prayers, become altars for the artists and the audience. They are created to invite the presence of a deity to cure individuals and restore a beneficial order for all. In sacred performances, such as those in the Luvale and Chewa cultures of Africa, dancers may become vehicles for the divinities of their tradition (Phiri, 2008; Nthala, 2011). Wearing the costumes and masks of deific beings increases the loss of individual identities in the dancers and promotes an experience of divine possession. This communicates intimations of the numinous to an audience in a receptive creative trance.

Tibetan dancing monks, also costumed and masked, make sacred sounds and symbolic gestures that are the culmination of extensive contemplative practices. The Tibetan tradition believes that seeing these dances and hearing the sacred music extends the wisdom of inner liberation to a lay audience steeped in the culture (Ricard, 2003). For Tibetan Buddhists, a sacred audience creative trance can bring freedom from the bondage of negative emotional states that prevent the attainment of inner peace.

Current electronic media has extended the reach of sacred settings. Now trance states can be generated in audiences far beyond the physical presence of the performers. When Fatna, a woman living in Rabat, heard music on television by the Gnawa, who are Moroccan ritual healers, she entered a deep trance (Kapchan, 2007). This happened although the television was playing in another room, and Fatma did not see images of the musicians but only heard their percussive music. Yet she felt that her trance, although unexpected, was a welcome experience and a profound link to the spiritual world.

CHAPTER 2

Consciousness and Creativity Theory in the Creative Trance

The quality of your consciousness at this moment is what shapes the future
Eckhart Tolle

The mind loves the unknown

Rene Magritte

Creativity, an apex of consciousness, contains the creative trance with its altered states that are treasured across cultures and time. Ranging from nostalgic reveries that can inspire great works of fiction, to the everyday creativity that enhances our lives, to the fast-moving action of sports that shape and reshape personal goals, the creative trance can also be a transcendent experience, an ecstasy using the body's own pharmacology. Yet consciousness is more easily experienced than defined and may possibly range from the galactically large to the microbiologically small.

Consciousness, Altered States of Consciousness, and the Creative Trance

Deriving from the Latin verb *conscire*, the word *consciousness* means to know or be aware of something, and as ordinary waking consciousness, it is the subjective awareness of ourselves, our existence, and our intentions (Krippner, 1999a). Recent research (Demertzi et al., 2019) has uncovered a neurological signature for human ordinary waking consciousness, yet the exact nature of consciousness remains elusive, although it may be pervasive. Hunt (1995) believes consciousness might be around us and within us, and we do not see it, as fish do not see the water in which they swim. There also appears to be a nonlocal aspect to consciousness (Di Biase, 2009; Schwartz, 2010, 2018; Murphy, 2019). Evidence for this is suggested by the effects of remote intercessory prayers (Dossey, 1993). Quantified studies on the efficacy of prayer indicate there can be benefits for human cancer patients (Olver & Dutney, 2012) and for nonhuman primates (Lesniak, 2006).

Scientists have found intimations of consciousness ranging from the intergalactically enormous to the microscopically minute. The astrophysicist Greg Matloff (2016) investigates minded or volitional stars, which appear to regulate their galactic trajectories through unipolar jets of stellar emissions, while the microbiologists Lynn Margulis and Barbara McClintock find indications of consciousness at the cellular level (Keller, 1983; Feldman, 2018). McClintock says that cells arrange their genomes in a sentient manner and Margulis believes that unicellular organisms respond consciously to their environment through the choices they make.

Existing somewhere on a spectrum between these enormously large and extremely small carriers of consciousness is the phenomenon of human consciousness. The American Psychological Association (APA) (2020) defines human consciousness as a waking state with an awareness that there is something either external or internal to oneself. Krippner (1997) further defines consciousness as an organism's continuing stream of cognition, affect, perception, and motivation. For Combs (2002, p. 7), consciousness is "the essence of experience … the perfect transparent subjectivity through which the phenomenal world shines. Without it, knowledge is only information."

Altered States of Consciousness

APA (2020) defines trance as an altered state of consciousness. If consciousness is our ongoing state of awareness, then an altered state of consciousness is an experience of psychological functioning significantly different from ordinary waking states (James, 1929; Tart, 1990; APA, 2020). Varying according to the individual, these states are often associated with transformed orientations about time and place, and can have different levels of self-awareness, reality testing, and response to stimuli. Some of these states may contain sensations of boundlessness, ecstasy, or union with the universe, becoming memorable experiences.

Altered states of consciousness include the creative process, meditations, hypnosis, reveries, prayer, dreams, and the hypnogogic or hypnopompic states between wakefulness and sleep. They may also arise from mystical experiences, religious ceremonies, or changed neurobiological functioning due to psychoactive drugs, sensory deprivation, or oxygen depletion. Although classical psychoanalysis regards altered states as psychologically regressive, humanistic psychology, Jungian psychology, and transpersonal psychology view them as elevated states of consciousness that may indicate a more advanced stage of personal and spiritual development (APA, 2020).

The Altered State of Relinquishing Control in the Creative Trance

In some instances of the creative trance there is an altered state of consciousness, which manifests as a willing loss of conscious control over the work produced. This dissociative experience, which will be discussed further in Chapters 3 and 4, can occur when individuals both acknowledge and voluntarily accept a loss of conscious decision-making during their creative process. At this point, the ego appears to willingly relinquish control to what is perceived to be the autonomy of the work. As the pianist Rosalyn Tureck (1913–2003) insisted, "I do what Bach tells me to do. I never tell the music what to do; I never make the decision; it – the music – makes the decision" (cited in Mach, 1991, p. 169). The singer, musician, and songwriter Stevie Wonder (Stevland Hardaway Morris, b. 1950), who sees his songs as a divine blessing, says, "I'm only being used as a vehicle" (cited in Rowden, 2012, pp. 115–116), "through which comes encouragement, inspiration, hope, and some clarity . . . . It is an honor to do it and I never forget the honor."

For writers, the loss of autonomy may include a temporary lapse in consensual reality. This can happen when the characters in their books seem to come alive and determine the course of the narrative. When the writer Alice Walker (b. 1944) was working on her novel *The Color Purple*, she said its characters complained and told her they did not like living in Brooklyn. So, she moved to San Francisco, but they did not like it there either (Currey, 2019). Finally, after renting a small cottage in Boonville, Northern California, which was more like the rural setting of the novel, they became friendly and talkative again. Walker said (cited in Currey, 2019 p. 118), "We would sit wherever I was sitting and talk. They were very obliging, engaging, and jolly."

Multiple Depths of a Creative Trance: The Lighter States

Like the altered states of the hypnotic trance, which the APA (2020) defines as having three levels, such as light, medium, and deep, the altered state of the creative trance also appears to have differing levels of depth. In its lighter manifestations, the creative trance would correspond to what Csikszentmihalyi (1990, 1996) defines as the state of flow, a time of enjoyable motivation, relaxation, and concentration on a task, where skills match challenges and goals are clear. Self-consciousness lessens as do sounds and distractions from the outside world, allowing the creative person to focus on the work. A light creative trance can occur during our everyday creativity, the originality we demonstrate throughout our daily life (Richards, 2018).

A widespread example of a light creative trance is doodling, with its small, quickly created visuals such as images, words, or abstract designs that require minimal concentration. Grosso (1997, p. 182), who connects creativity with dissociation, notes that "the dissociative process is a matter of degree," and cites doodling as an activity with a light state of dissociation. What he identifies as a light state of dissociation appears to correspond to a light state of creative trance. Although Grosso notes that doodling can progress to automatic writing or drawing, which indicates deeper states of trance, it usually remains a light, pleasurable short-term experience.

Doodling is so prevalent and enjoyable that even the humanist scholar Erasmus (Desiderius Erasmus Roterodamus, 1466–1536) doodled on his writings. Stewart (2013, p. 409) calls Erasmus a "habitual doodler" and says he "often made figurative scribbles . . . in the margins of his books." Erasmus, who did manuscript decoration in his youth, created numerous doodles on his work, including a self-portrait in the form of a mask on his 1515 document the *Epistles of Saint Jerome*. Although doodling constitutes a light creative trance, it has a noticeable effect on brain chemistry. Using functional near-infrared spectroscopy Kaimala and associates (2017) found that doodling, even more than freehand drawing or coloring in already created designs, maximized blood flow to the medial prefrontal cortex, a reward center in the brain.

With concentration, the light creative trance of an everyday creativity can evolve into a deeper state. The choreographer and artistic director of the New York City Ballet George Balanchine (1904–1983) took delight in everyday creativity. He liked cooking but refused to purchase a food processor because he enjoyed chopping food (Austen, 2013). Balanchine also preferred to do his own laundry, and had a portable washing machine installed in his New York apartment (Currey, 2014). But what he liked best was ironing, an activity that stimulated his creative thinking. "When I'm ironing," he said, "that's when I do most of my work" (cited in Currey, 2014 p. 124). Balanchine took an activity associated with a light creative trance, and through concentrated creativity, transformed it into a medium creative trance that generated his choreography.

Multiple Depths of a Creative Trance: The Medium States

Jane Austen (1775–1817), Agatha Christie (1890–1976), and E. B. White (1899–1985) provide examples of a medium creative trance because they all wrote at home during the activities of daily life (Plimpton, 1988; Christie, 2010). Austen and White wrote in their living rooms with people coming in and out, while Christie worked on any surface solid enough to support a typewriter, including her washstand in the bedroom and her dining room table between meals. Yet Christie said the times when she was able to be uninterrupted in a room with a closed door were her most productive. Then she could write more quickly, becoming lost in her work.

Another example of a medium state of creative trance is the experience of the primatologist Jane Goodall (b. 1934), but here stimuli from the outside world do not diminish. Instead, they amplify and augment the creative trance. Goodall recalls a sense of wonder and awe while working in Tanzania with chimpanzees in Gombe National Park. It had been pouring rain, but suddenly the rain stopped, and Goodall said (cited in Zetlin, 2018, n.p.), "I could smell the wet hair on the chimpanzees, and I could hear the insects singing loudly, and I just felt absolutely at one."

Multiple Depths of a Creative Trance: Deeper States

In a deep creative trance, the person is profoundly immersed and focused on work, to the exclusion of everything else. Sounds and distractions from the outside world completely cease to exist. Some individuals in a deep creative trance may also be in a state of hyperfocus (see Chapter 8 for a discussion of hyperfocus). No matter what else may be happening at that moment, during a deep creative trance the entire universe consists only of the creative person and the work in progress. Jack Snow (1943–2006), who played football for the Los Angeles Rams, provides evidence of a deep creative trance. He describes this experience as intense concentration and a form of self-hypnosis, saying (cited in Murphy & White, 1995, p. 23), "If a plane crashed in the stadium, I don't think I'd notice it until the play was over."

The Italian Renaissance artist Francesco Mazzuola (1503–1540), known as Parmigianino, provides another example of a deep creative trance. One day in 1527, Parmigianino was so engrossed in his work that he did not hear the tumultuous events taking place in the street outside his home (Vasari, 1996). It was the Sack of Rome, and German armies were invading the city. Extremely absorbed in painting, Parmigianino noticed absolutely nothing of the exterior world until German soldiers were already in his studio. Fortunately, the soldiers were so impressed with his art that they left him unharmed.

Absorption and the Depths of a Creative Trance

The degree of depth in a creative trance depends on multiple factors, including the time and place of the creative activity, the importance of the creative work to the person engaged in it, the emotional state of the creative person, and the presence of a psychological tendency known as *absorption*. Increasing levels of absorption, which is the capacity to be immersed in something, appear to correspond with aspects of the medium and especially the deeper states of a creative trance. The propensity for absorption shows a strong correlation with hypnotizability (Tellegen & Atkinson, 1974) and may have some congruence with the experience of hyperfocus in ADHD (Gaev, 2021). Glisky and associates (1991) find absorption has a connection to creativity through its propensity for imagery, dreams, and fantasy, which are aspects of the personality trait of openness to experience.

Absorption, which appears to be an experience of trance, takes place, as Tellegen and Atkinson (1974) note, in an altered state of consciousness. Using the Tellegen Absorption Scale, a self-report questionnaire, Tellegen and Atkinson (1974, p. 274) found that people with a disposition for absorption can experience "total attention." This highly focused altered state commandeers all a person's perceptual, imaginative, ideational, and motoric resources to concentrate on the object of their attention. In response, the person becomes impervious to distractions, while the attentional object, whether it is an image, a work of art, a piece of music, a memory, or a fantasy, acquires an intensified reality.

For some, the experience of absorption in early life may be a creative trance that sets the course of an adult career (Zausner, 2016). During his isolation from the family due to tuberculosis in childhood, the sculptor Tony Smith (1912–1980) would focus on the most important piece of furniture in his room, a black metal stove. Smith stared at the stove until it became "a little god" (cited in Storr, 1998, p. 12). As a mature artist, Smith created large geometric sculptures, often in black metal like the stove of his childhood.

When the visual artist Max Ernst (1891–1976) was sick with measles in childhood, he stared at the false mahogany pattern on furniture by his bed until its lines began to alter before his eyes, creating a changing variety of shapes (Rossalbi, 1975). In adulthood, changing forms and altered images became central to his surrealist paintings. Absorption can also bring benefits to musical performance. As a young pianist, Rosalind Tureck (1913–2003) entered a competition and was so absorbed in the music that she remembers nothing from the time she sat down to play until the bell rang to stop (Mach, 1991). Yet Tureck's performance was so excellent that she was awarded a diamond medal.

Everyday Creativity and the Creative Trance

Creativity, the guiding force of great art and personal growth, also exists as an everyday creative trance, the altered state of consciousness fundamental to the everyday creativity of daily life (Montuori et al., 2004; Richards, 2018). All our problem-solving activity is creative, ranging from the small solutions that improve our life to the life-changing decisions that transform it. Every choice we make is a creative determination, a response to multiple variables generating projections for the future. During those times preceding choice, when possibilities are considered, outcomes are weighed, trajectories are compared, and decisions are planned, we are in an everyday creative trance. Varying from seconds to hours and ranging greatly in complexity, it is central to survival in our multifaceted existence.

The creative trance of everyday life takes various forms and may happen multiple times per day. Gardening, arranging items for aesthetic or useful purposes, fixing what has been broken, and all our instances of daily problem-solving are its many facets. These moments of trance in daily life become treasured temporal vacations from the larger expanse of ordinary waking awareness. They are a time away from our usual time and, through their separateness and their focus, they can become experiences of relief, relaxation, and accomplishment.

The Everyday Creative Trance as a Culturally Mediated Experience

The everyday creative trance can arise during work or whenever we are focused on a task. It may occur in those moments of happy fulfillment when work is going well, but may also happens when the situation is frustrating, and we persevere despite the frustrations. Just as our lives are shaped by the societies in which we live, so can our everyday trance be a culturally mediated experience. We see this in the following two examples of a work-related creative trance, one from Australia and the other from Canada.

Australian Aborigine people have produced some of the worlds most accomplished trackers. Tracking animals for sustenance in a harsh climate is a survival skill learned in childhood and further honed as an adult. It appears to have its own type of altered state. For some trackers, the creative trance can be a time of deliberate movements until a realization occurs. When the well-known tracker Mitamirri (c.1902–1945) was asked how he worked (cited in Sevilla, 2019, n.p.) he said, "I never bend down low, just walk slow round and round until I see more."

The Canadian psychologist Imants Barušs (b. 1952) describes his total involvement while lecturing as a pleasurable work state. "I become absorbed in drawing on my knowledge of the subject matter and organizing it into a narrative structure," says Barušs (2003, p. 188). "The usual concerns of everyday life disappear into the background, and I lose track of time," Barušs compares his experience to Csikszentmihalyi's (1990, 1996) concept of flow. The state of flow, which encompasses immersion and enjoyment in an activity, setting goals, reduced awareness of outside distractions, and the passage of time, has great congruence with the state of a light creative trance.

Theories of Creativity and the Creative Trance: Habitual Responses and Divergent Thinking

Originality enlivens the creative process, both for the creator and the audience. Barron (1969) believes that the propensity to originality tends to be habitual in the lives of creative people. He suggests that creative individuals have ongoing patterns of response to experience, which become a precondition for their consistent creativity. An aspect of this habitual response to experience may be the tendency for creative people to engage in divergent thinking. This type of thinking, which produces numerous and diverse solutions to a problem, is generally intuitive, automatic, associative, and diffuse (Gabora & Kaufman, 2010).

In its capacity to generate multiple new and creative solutions, divergent thinking also includes bravery to face the unusual and a willingness to accept change. We see these capacities in two quotes by Albert Einstein: "If, at first, the idea is not absurd, then there is no hope for it," and "We cannot solve problems by using the same kind of thinking we used when we created them" (cited in Hickman & Banister, 2005, p. 24).

Theories of Creativity and the Creative Trance: Five Factor Model and Openness

Why some people tend to think in a divergent manner and are habitually more creative than others leads to research on the five factor model of personality, comprised of neuroticism, extraversion, agreeableness, conscientiousness, and openness (Goldberg, 1993; Bagby et al., 2005; Widiger & Costa, 2012). In this taxonomy of personality traits, openness is identified with creativity and its allied aspects including divergent thinking, imagination, intellect, curiosity, unconventionality, and flexibility.

An individual high in openness is the type of person most likely to enter a creative trance. Yet like the other four personality traits, openness has maladaptive variants, which are the extremes of the trait. A person very low in openness would tend to be rigid, superficial, and not prone to creativity, while someone overly high in openness would tend to be unrealistic and might be lost in fantasy. People overly high in openness could enter a trance state but may have difficulties translating their visions into concrete form.

Kaufman and associates (2016) found that openness to experience predicts artistic achievement while openness to intellect predicts creativity in science. They also found a connection between extraversion and artistic creativity but not with creativity in science. Wolfradt and Pretz (2001) postulate there is an eventual progression from extraversion to introversion as an individual attains proficiency in a domain. They believe that while social interaction may initially stimulate creativity, it takes concerted solitary effort to bring creative ideas into fruition and reach a level of expertise.

Theories of Creativity and the Creative Trance: Its Levels and Sudden Insights

An additional theory of creativity examines its levels of expression from everyday creativity, known as little-c, to eminent creativity, known as Big-C (Merrotsy, 2013; Kozbelt et al., 2019). This division is further delineated into four levels of creative achievement by Kaufman and Beghetto (2009). Their first level, mini-c creativity, is inherent in everyday creativity, while at the second level, little-c creativity, everyday creative accomplishments are valued by others. The third or Pro-c level is professional creative accomplishment after years of training, and the fourth or Big-C level of creativity is the attainment of historically recognized eminence. The creative trance is present in all four levels of creativity, but may vary from a light, to a medium, to a deep trance, depending on the level of commitment, intensity of work, and working methods of the creative person.

Wallas' (1926) four-stage model of the creative process, consisting of preparation, incubation, illumination, and verification, has a creative trance in the first, third, and fourth stages, but it is the third stage, illumination that contains one of the most dramatic occurrences of a creative trance. Here, content from the unconscious mind suddenly erupts into conscious awareness as a problem-solving insight that becomes the dominant reality for the length of the trance. Among the people Wallas used to illustrate the appearance of sudden insights was the mathematician Henri Poincare (1854–1912), who wrote about these insights in his essay *Mathematical Creation* (Poincare, 2000).

It was when Poincare was working on one of his earliest discoveries, Fuchsian functions (preparation), and not consciously thinking about the mathematics (incubation), that he had four experiences of insight (illumination) that solved previously difficult problems in his computations (verification). The first insight came after a sleepless night when crowds of ideas collided in his mind, yet by morning they had combined into the geometry of the Fuchsian functions. The second insight into the Fuchsian functions came while he was boarding a bus to a geological site and the third while he was walking on a bluff by the sea, both excursions to get his mind off the frustrations of work. The fourth insight came while walking down a street in Mont-Valérian, where he went for military service. In all instances, Poincare (2000, p. 98) transcribed his insights into mathematical form (verification) and said that with each of them there was a "feeling of absolute certitude accompanying the inspiration."

The Creative Trance as a Pivot to Transformation

Prevalent throughout humanity, the creative trance is an altered state of consciousness that we enter naturally when we are creative. In its myriad forms across domains, it is fundamental to the creative process, and evident from prehistoric cultures to the current day. A fluid state, filled with possibilities, the creative trance can be a time of power and a pivot point of change in life. When contents of the unconscious mind become more accessible to conscious awareness, multiple options appear, allowing us to transform our work and ourselves. Then the creative trance becomes an experience of transformation, because by changing ourselves, we can change our world (Zausner, 2016).

When the pivot point in a creative trance contains an epiphany, it can elicit a profound transformation of consciousness, as it did for the photographer Mariette Pathy Allen (b. 1940). In 1978, on holiday with her husband for the Mardi Gras in New Orleans, Allen (2021) met a group of cross-dressers staying at her hotel. They were very friendly and as Pathy started to photograph one of them, she said (Allen, 2021, online), "So, I lifted the camera to my eye and, looking through the lens ... I said to myself – it just came to me – I'm not looking at a man or a woman, I'm looking at a human being. I'm looking at a soul." After New Orleans, Pathy continued photographing the cross-dressing population and had a second epiphany. "Suddenly," she said, "I realized I'd been given a huge gift. I began to feel like I was the conduit through which information could be disseminated about people who had been degraded." Pathy became an advocate for gender variance, whose recent book (Allen, 2017) is about the gender-fluid spirit mediums living in Burma and Thailand.

The Creative Trance: Its Clinical and Social Aspects and Its Capacity for Transcendence

The creative trance can play a central role in clinical work. Trance states, such as those in hypnosis and the inner processing and visualization of EMDR, are basic to clinical practice in its quest to recreate the self as a more highly functioning being. Psychological theory has also addressed the clinical aspects of transcendent states as steps in self-evolution. Carl Jung (1971) called them numinous, William James (1929) characterized them as mystic consciousness, while for Maslow (1964) they were peak experiences. The quest for transcendence and its concept of an extended non-corporeal self is evident in Paleolithic funerary objects suggesting that metaphysical beliefs are ancient and possibly inherent in human consciousness. These beliefs are now studied as quantified experiments in contemporary post-materialist psychology (Beauregard et al., 2018). Correlating theories are found in rites of initiation (Eliade, 1965, 1975) and in the psychology of shamanism (Krippner, 2002; Winkelman, 2011).

The creative trance, usually a positive experience, can have negative aspects when individuals abuse alcohol and drugs to facilitate creativity, sometimes with deleterious consequences (Zausner, 2011a). Anxiety from phobias may also block creative expression. When fear of speaking in public inhibits the creative trance of oration, it deprives both speaker and audience of a potentially positive event. Another negative aspect is malevolent creativity, when the creative process is intentionally used for harmful results (Cropley et al., 2008; Harris et al., 2013).

The Shared Creative Trance: Enjoyment, Synchronization, and Cultural Transmission

A very enjoyable aspect of the creative trance is that it can be shared. Just as it is normal to be in and out of altered states throughout daily life, therefore shared altered states are also a normal part of existence. There is the shared trance of an audience in rapt attention, riveted on a performance, and the group concentrating and listening together to poems or stories. There is also a unifying shared trance with the emergent synchronization of clapping in applause or in rhythmic accompaniment to music. There are the mutual interactive trance states of partners dancing and singing and the trance connecting a group of dancers and singers both secular and spiritual. When the creative trance is a shared trance, it can promote social coherence and cultural transmission.

Twele, a contemporary Kalahari Bushman, says that in his society dance is "our prayer, our medicine, our teaching, and our way of having fun. Everything we do is related to that dance" (cited in Heeney, 2005, p. 49). With its capacity for intrabrain and interbrain synchronization, dance promotes enjoyment, personal growth, and social relations (Basso et al., 2021). The entrainment and motor synchrony of dance may be an indicator of kinesthetic empathy and possibly associated with oxytocin, a neurotransmitter and hormone linked to affiliation and empathic connections (Josef et al., 2019). The emergent synchronization of reciprocal entrainment is now being charted by social neuroscience, yielding data that may support the concept of a shared creative trance.

The Shared Creative Trance: Neural Synchronization and Extended Consciousness

Just as the emergence of each cognitive moment within one brain relies on a synchrony of oscillations among widespread brain regions (Varela et al., 2001; Strogatz, 2003), so may the coordinated behavior of separate brains exhibit a neural synchronization (Valencia & Froese, 2020). This synchrony of interpersonal coordination and mutual entrainment suggests an emergent order (Czeszumski et al., 2020) in the ongoing emergence of consciousness (Feinberg & Mallatt, 2020). The intention toward cooperation in a shared creative trance may be conscious or unconscious, but the neural synchronization appears to be driven by the unconscious mind.

Synchronized states can be mapped by hyperscanning, a neuroimaging technique that studies and evaluates electronic data received from multiple brains simultaneously (Czeszumski et al., 2020). It can discern neural synchrony in activities that this book would identify as having a shared creative trance. These synchronized activities can include performing music together (Acquadro et al., 2016), singing (Osaka et al., 2015), jointly solving puzzles (Fishburn et al., 2018), and participating in cooperative games (De Vico Fallani et al., 2010). Investigations of interbrain synchronization during group dynamics (Szymanski et al., 2017) found that certain individuals work more easily together than others, recommending that this measure of social facilitation might be useful in explaining why some teams are more successful.

Humans are social beings, who tend to produce emergent order through interactions with each other (Acquadro et al., 2016). Influencing other consciousnesses and being influenced by them in return (Basso et al., 2021) intimates intersubjectivity and a deep capacity for connection. By studying the neural basis of these relationships, social neuroscience is now proposing that consciousness may not only be an individual experience but also a shared experience (Basso et al., 2021). Supporting this concept are the numerous connections within one brain and between brains that might be regarded as hyper brain networks (De Vico Fallani et al., 2010). Current research suggests (Froese & Fuchs, 2012; Froese et al., 2013; Valencia & Froese, 2020) that neural hyperconnectivity may provide a window into the interactive facet of human cognition, implying the possibility of expanded consciousness and the prospect of an extended mind.

CHAPTER 3

Unconscious Origins of the Creative Trance

Civilization advances by extending the number of important operations which we can perform without thinking about them
Alfred North Whitehead

The brain is wider than the sky
Emily Dickinson

We live in a multiplicity of personal worlds, all connected through the power of our unconscious mind and its capacity for trance. There is the world of our waking life, the world of our reveries, the world of our sleeping dreams, and the world we enter when we are creative. Waking life is the purview of conscious thought shaped by unconscious motivations, while reveries are the daydreams that give form to unconscious desires. Dreams during sleep are the poetry of the unconscious mind and creativity is a shifting amalgam of conscious and unconscious thinking. Whenever we connect to the unconscious in our personal worlds it becomes possible to experience trance. As an altered state of consciousness opening directly into the capacities of the unconscious mind, trance is pervasive in our lives.

The Unconscious Mind

Yet what is this neural vastness we call the unconscious mind? Significantly larger than the conscious mind, it influences most of our thoughts, emotions, and actions (Bargh, 2005). Fluid and capable of expansion, its internal aspects of mind affect our conscious thinking and behavior, although they are not conscious themselves (Uleman, 2005). The unconscious, as source and director of creative output, is highly active during creativity and its states of trance. Two disciplines that focus on unconscious functioning are clinical psychology and cognitive psychology (APA, 2020). Cognitive psychology investigates the unconscious processes and mental structures of an individual (Kihlstrom, 1987). These aspects include the perceptual-cognitive abilities, automated motor skills, and implicit memories that facilitate creative expression. In clinical psychology, the unconscious is a repository of material including desires, memories, repressed impulses, and emotional conflicts that are hidden from conscious awareness to avoid shame, anxiety, or guilt. Yet this consciously unknowable emotional content (APA, 2020) drives the inspiration and passion of a creative trance.

The creative trance is profoundly open to unconscious influence. We are creatures of the unconscious and we are fortunate because the unconscious is vast. Its control over our mental processes and our lives gives us greater and deeper experiences than would be possible through the more limited conscious mind alone. Access to the unconscious and its influence appear to operate on a spectrum ranging from the daily decisions of everyday life, which usually carry a sense of conscious intention, to the wider more amorphous states of the creative trance, where unconscious processes openly influence conscious behavior. The unconscious is everywhere beneath the veneer of the conscious mind. Like our planet, where the visible is grounded in the unseen, waking consciousness would be the mountains and outcroppings of rocks, whose origins go deep into the earth, corresponding to the hidden depth of the unconscious mind.

The Unconscious Mind: Its History and Structures

The concept of an unconscious aspect of mind dates from antiquity. Dehaene (2014) finds acknowledgments of unconscious control in ancient Greece and Rome with the writings of Hippocrates, Galen, Plotinus, and Augustine. He notes that the eleventh-century Arab scientist Alhazen and the nineteenth-century German scientist von Helmholtz both used the term "unconscious inference" (p. 50), and that Spinoza, Descartes, and Leibniz also wrote that human behaviors and emotions derive from a hidden source. In the nineteenth and twentieth centuries, the unconscious mind became a focus of mainstream clinical study (Ellenberger, 1970). It included the work of Charcot, Bernheim, Janet, Adler, and Ferenczi among others, and the widely read writings of Freud and Jung.

In Freudian mental topography (Freud, 1963/1915), the unconscious mind is divided into the preconscious, with material that is potentially available to consciousness, and the unconscious, a storehouse of memories, urges, and desires. Although latent, they direct our thoughts and behaviors, generating both dreams and art. Jung (1969) divides the unconscious mind into a personal unconscious, specific to an individual, and the collective unconscious, a deep substrate of mind that all humans share. The collective unconscious contains archetypes, which are non-physical essences that appear to us as archetypal symbols or images in religions, dreams, and works of art. Influencing our emotions, thoughts, and actions, archetypal images have a similar meaning across cultures and time.

Nonclinical research in cognitive psychology also focuses on the unconscious mind. Kihlstrom (1987) calls it the cognitive unconscious, and postulates a three-part organization comprised of the preconscious, the subconscious, and the completely unconscious. Kihlstrom finds the unconscious is the repository of processes such as declarative knowledge and innate capacities that operate completely outside of conscious awareness. Functions such as nonautomated procedural knowledge and implicit memory are part of the preconscious, while the subconscious contains hypnosis and related dissociative states. The actions and capacities of the cognitive unconscious are the engines that facilitate the creative process.

The Cognitive Unconscious: Its Processes and Connection to Creativity

The cognitive unconscious is the part of our mind that processes unreportable mental activities, such as perception, thoughts, habits, and language (APA, 2020). It also carries out complex behaviors, motor actions, and planning, which are activities that through practice and repetition can become automated skills encoded in implicit memory (Bargh, 2005; Kihlstrom, 2008). Without entering our conscious awareness, these proficiencies become the unconscious abilities of fluid expertise. Rapidly executed without great effort or intention, automatic processes show major reductions of cortical activity in neuroimaging (APA, 2020). Playing musical scales becomes automated behavior as does learning a sequence of connected moves in dance, figure skating, and high diving. Incorporated in sequence as implicit memory, automatic behaviors become tools for achieving a goal of excellence. We see this in the violinist who no longer consciously concentrates on finger positions while playing, the ballet dancer who can perform a leap without halting deliberation, and the archer who can instinctually position a bow.

Implicit Motor Memory: Painting without Looking

The motor skills of implicit memory may also be able to resolve problems in a painting that elude the watchful eye and more consciously controlled hand. As Jung (2014, CW-8:180) remarked, "Often the hands know how to solve a riddle with which the intellect has wrestled in vain." This was my personal experience while working on a large oil painting called *Memories* (Zausner, 2011b). It was very late at night and I had been struggling for hours, painting and repainting clouds in an overcast sky, but getting nowhere. Finally, in sheer frustration, I could no longer bear to look at the canvas with its exasperating clouds, but neither was I able to stop working.

So, I painted without looking, my face turned away from the image, and only periodically looked down at the palette to load my brush with pigment. Finally, after some time of painting without looking, I faced the canvas and there was the structure of the clouds that I wanted but could not get before. My hand and arm painted them without my eyes. All the forms were created as a strong underpainting, and only needed the richness of glazing that brings depth and nuance to an image. Had I tried to paint the delicacy of a face without looking, I do not think it would have been as successful. Yet with the broad swaths of cloud structure, my implicit motor memories could paint what my conscious direction was not able to accomplish.

The Unconscious Mind: A Creative Dialectic in the Creative Trance

For most people, there is dialectic in the creative process and its trance states that advances the work forward through a series of iterations. This dialectic forms through the multiple and reciprocal efforts that bring the imagined products of creativity into a shareable reality. It consists of visualizations that inspire the work, which change in response to the progressing work, while the work changes in response to the sequence of altered visualizations. This ongoing dialectic of reciprocal responses produces a series of iterations that continue until the work is finished and the goal is met.

There may also be a dialectic between the conscious and the unconscious mind in the creative trance. We can only know the conscious half of this dialectic exchange, yet we might assume that an unconscious aspect also exists. Possibly, the sequential fleeting inspirations or decisions in the creative process may suggest this type of interaction. When a series of conscious thoughts appear to evolve consecutively with short spaces between them, we might infer that in the unheard or unknown spaces between the consciously received ideas may be the unconscious part of a dialectic exchange.

The Cognitive Unconscious: Multiple Variables and Parallel Processing

Creativity is a harmonic of many notes, brought together in a synthesis greater than the sum of its parts. Its creative depth exists as a blend of inspiration and originality, fused with training, tradition, expertise, and implicit memory, which are colored by emotions, past events, the environment, and the moment of creation, all generated by an individual with a lifetime of skill and experience. These multiple variables can interact quickly and without conscious awareness, because according to parallel distributed processing theory, the unconscious mind is a very fast parallel processor (Kihlstrom, 1987; Hunt, 1995).

Unlike the slow sequential thinking of the conscious mind, the unconscious can process numerous items that simultaneously influence and interact with each other facilitating a rapid analysis and synthesis of information. Parallel processing brings an unconsciously layered depth and complexity to the creative process and its product. The audience respond to this richness with a storehouse of experience and expectations generated by their own unconscious parallel processes. Unconscious parallel processing is basic to the complexity of the creative trance where multiple variables generate layers of depth in works of art.

This is evident in the painter who immediately knows what colors, brushes, and brushstrokes to use when painting a tree by unconsciously comparing the tree on the canvas to other trees he has created, to his training in landscape painting, and to the myriad trees he has seen in his lifetime. It is evident in the actor who empathically blends herself into a character by unconsciously harnessing her past experiences of multiple other roles and years of training and life events, and then fuses them into the current storyline of the script. It is also evident in a writer who creates a character that he consciously believes is a blend of two people he knows. Yet unconsciously, the character is an amalgam of multiple people he has met in his lifetime with similarities to the person in his text along with his responses to them and the memories of their various encounters. Although

the painter, the actor, and the writer may think they are working consciously, the greater part of their choices and the causal engines of their
expertise come from parallel processing in the unconscious mind.

The Unconscious Mind: Illusions of Conscious Control and Free Will

We do not know that moment or millisecond when we enter unconscious
control. The borderline between conscious and unconscious functioning is
blurred and liminal, unapparent to waking awareness. We cross that
boundary countless times in daily life. The frequency and ease of this
transition facilitates the trance state during creativity, yet current experimental research indicates that the unconscious mind also controls our daily
decisions. Previously, the unconscious was a less recognized force behind
everyday behavior, but now it increasingly reveals its dominant role.

In a set of well-known neurophysiology studies, Libet and associates
(1993; Libet, 1999) demonstrated that conscious intention is not the initial
cause of our actions. Instead, they found that the unconscious initiates
most of our movements and choices although we may believe they are
conscious decisions. By measuring neural activity in response to the decision to move a finger, Libet and associates discovered that an electrical shift
in the brain called the readiness potential (RP) precedes physical movement by 550 milliseconds. When they asked subjects to check a clock for
the time of their conscious decision to move a finger, it was about 350 to
400 milliseconds after the recorded RP in the brain, demonstrating that the
impetus to motion begins in the unconscious mind. These experiments
suggest some of the ways that unconscious functioning dominates motor
processes during the creative trance even though there may be a feeling of
conscious control.

While acknowledging the dominance of the unconscious, Libet (1999)
also addresses the existence of free will. He finds that conscious control can
veto unconscious action if a conscious decision, such as not to move
a finger, occurs about 200 milliseconds before movement is begun. Libet
says that while free will could not begin a voluntary action, it could control
its outcome or performance. This indicates that in creativity, we can stop
or amend actions generated by the unconscious if the conscious mind
believes they should be altered. Because of our capacity to override unconscious actions, Libet believes we have free will and advocates for his
position by quoting the writer Isaac Bashevis Singer (1902–1991). Singer
states (cited in Libet, 1999, p. 56), "The greatest gift which humanity has

received is free choice. It is true that we are limited in our use of free choice. But the little free choice we have is such a great gift and is potentially worth so much that for this itself life is worthwhile living."

The Unconscious Mind: Illusions of Control and Responsibility

The reaches of the unconscious blur when they meet the conscious mind, resulting not only in the illusion of conscious control but also, under certain circumstances, in a tendency to assume responsibility for actions initiated by someone else. In another set of well-known experiments Wegner and Wheatley (1999) demonstrated this when they paired two people at a board game who shared a cursor to select images on a computer screen. One person was the research subject, and the other person, unbeknownst to the research subject, was a confederate of the experimenters. Both the research subject and the confederate wore headphones and were informed they would hear music and words, but the confederate was also given instructions about which image to select.

Wegner and Wheatley found that when the subjects heard a word in their headphones that matched an image on the screen one to five seconds before the confederate forced the cursor to that image, the subjects felt it was they who choose the image. If the word was given thirty seconds prior or one second after the choice of image, it generated a smaller sense of personal intention. These experiments reveal that under certain circumstances we can be prone to claim conscious control over actions that are not our own. Wegner and Wheatley find the belief that actions originate in our conscious mind to be an error based on the illusion of will. Instead, they state (Wegner & Wheatley, 1999, p. 492) that "the real causes of human action are unconscious."

Bargh (2005, p. 41) agrees, saying that the experience of conscious control is illusory because "causation is always an inference and never something directly observable." In the past researchers believed automatic and unconscious processes were the exception, but current cognitive psychology recognizes them as the norm and comprising most of our mentation, while conscious activity is now seen as the exception (Kihlstrom, 2008). Although we have an inherent bias to believe we consciously control our actions in reaching a goal, it appears instead that the conscious intention of striving toward a goal activates a sequence of unconscious motor movements.

This is a foundation of the creative trance and evident in the basketball player who consciously wants to score a basket, but whose physical actions come from implicit memories and skills encoded in his unconscious. It is also evident in improvisational jazz where the musician's fingers seem to choose the notes they play when her conscious awareness blends with the music generated by her band. The basketball player and the musician are examples of acceding to unconscious control and current cognitive science finds we are prone to unconscious control.

Acquiescing to Unconscious Control in the Creative Trance

We are also capable of completely voluntary movements that still feel unwilled. Called *neuropsychological anomalies* (Wegner & Wheatley, 1999, p. 482), they are instances where people are aware of their actions but feel they are engaging in them without conscious intention. These are the times during the creative process when people feel "things just happen." Motor actions, complex behaviors, and higher mental processes can all be initiated without conscious awareness, and Bargh (2005) believes that the human brain was constructed for such independence. Apparent across creative domains, energies from the unconscious appear without conscious volition, yet metamorphose into actions that can enhance a work in progress. This may be why creative individuals, who are already acclimated to unconscious control, willingly allow the unconscious to control them during the creative trance.

Acquiescing to the unconscious mind in the creative trance can produce unforeseen occurrences that greatly improve the work in ways not possible through conscious control. Creative people view them as beneficial "surprises." In these creative surprises, the unconscious completely dominates physical actions. Manifesting as movements that appear to "come out of nowhere," they are gifts of the creative trance. These are all the brushstrokes that were seemingly unintentional but bring the painting to a new level, all the unplanned dance moves that enhance a performance, and the direction a fictional character takes during writing that deviates from yet exceeds the previously planned script. Acknowledging the unconsciously metamorphic nature of creativity, the visual artist Marcel Duchamp (1887–1968) suggests there should be an art coefficient to compute the difference between what was originally intended by the creative person and what appears in the final work (Duchamp, 1973).

Unconscious creative interventions also make it easier to designate inspiration to outside sources. For Duchamp (1973, p. 138), the creative person is a "mediumistic being," and the visual artist Paul Klee (1879–1940) (1969, p. 15) saw himself as "merely a channel." The songwriter Carole King (b. 1942) believed that, "When the thing you're creating comes *through* you, you know it, and it's much better than good enough" (cited in Currey, 2019, p. 120). Retha Walden Gambaro, who created sculptures related to her Native American Cree tradition, felt a miraculous force controlling her hands when she worked and wondered, "How am I doing this?" (cited in Lacey, 2012).

Difficulties with Conscious and Unconscious Control in the Creative Trance

Conversely, in instances where creativity clings to conscious control, such as repeating works that were previously produced or copying the work of another person, the results can leave a staleness in the finished product. A work generated by the unconscious mind and shaped by its unforeseen surprises contains greater energy and originality, and communicates this to the audience.

There can also be unwanted consequences of unconscious control, such as the tendency in figurative artists to recreate their own faces in the people they paint. In his notebooks (1970a), Leonardo da Vinci (1452–1519) warns artists to be aware of this tendency and to correct it. Artists may also unconsciously recreate the faces of people they know on the figures they are painting. I have found this in my own work. At times, the faces of people I know will appear on a figure in my art without any conscious awareness that I am painting their likeness or even thinking about them. Presumably, although these individuals were completely hidden from my conscious mind, they were active enough in what Freud and Kihlstrom would identify as my preconscious to surface in a work of art.

The Unconscious, the Creative Trance, and Awareness without Volition

The role of the unconscious is central to the creative trance. A definition of trance that suggests its unconscious origins describes it as a state of awareness without the feeling of self-determination (Barušs, 2003). This seemingly paradoxical phenomenon occurs when a person who is actively creating willingly believes she is relinquishing her authority to the work in progress and accepts that the work controls what she creates. The experience of a creative work controlling the creator takes many forms. Friedrich Nietzsche (1844–1900) (2020/1911, p. 47) believes that "one hears – one does not seek; one takes – one does not ask... Everything happens quite involuntarily." The visual artist Joan Mitchell (1925–1992) says, "I sit and look at the painting, sometimes for hours. Eventually, the painting tells me what to do" (cited in Currey, 2019 p. 134).

Would it be advisable or even possible for a creative person to go against the wishes of her work in progress? I can attest from personal experience as a visual artist that for me it is neither advisable nor possible if one aims for the best creative results. My work tells me what to do, even if I do not agree. Once, I tried to push back against the will of a painting, but to no avail. I failed and the painting won. It happened when I was working on *The Pilgrim*, a large oil on canvas depicting a solitary figure carrying a burden while crossing a long narrow bridge that ended on land in the foreground. My intention was to paint a nice garden where he could rest, his journey over. The painting kept insisting on a road in the foreground, so the figure could continue walking. This made me angry because I wanted the figure to rest but none of the gardens I painted were acceptable in the composition. Finally, I gave in and painted the road. It was the best and only solution.

Projective Identification and an Unconscious Hierarchy of Power

Yet why would a creator become an employee of the work she creates? What would be a clinical explanation for this pervasive dictatorship in works of art? It may be possible that in a state of absorption, such as focused creativity, the work of art can act as an attentional object that grows in importance and autonomy (Tellegen & Atkinson, 1974). Ehrenzweig (1971), who notes that a work of art appears to have its own independent life, says (p. 102) that for artists it "acts like another living person with whom we are conversing." He identifies this experience as projective identification, which was further theorized by Melanie Klein. For Klein (1996) projective identification is an unconscious experience in which parts of the self are split-off and projected into an outside object. Klein warns about excessive splitting, saying the projected part can control the person who projects it.

While Klein pathologizes this state of control as unhealthy in interpersonal relations, in the creative process it appears to be a widespread and nonpathological experience. I call this occurrence an *artistic projection*. One is reminded of the statement by Kris (1971, p. 60), that in psychosis, "the ego is overwhelmed by the primary process," yet in art, "the ego controls the primary process and puts it into its service." Similarly, in interpersonal relationships, where projective identification may become a negative dissolution, during creativity, it can be used in the service of art.

A fusion of the artistic projection with a work of art appears to generate an unconscious hierarchy of power and control in the artist's mind, possibly akin to the establishment of a creative executive function now apparently located in the work in progress. A result may be the artist's acceptance of a seemingly outside authority that appears to know and communicate what needs to be done.

The projection occurrence is widespread in the creative trance and has aspects of both empathy and dissociation, which will be further discussed in Chapter 4. Like empathy, there is an intuitive awareness about the needs of another. Yet in this case the other is a work of art, and unlike empathy, there is a relinquishment of conscious creative control. It is also a partially dissociative state because the creative person unconsciously dissociates part of herself and projects it into the work in progress. The possibility and ease of unconscious projections may derive from what appears to be our pluralistic psychological nature.

The Parts Work of Ego State Therapy

According to the psychologists John Watkins and Helen Watkins (1997), we are multifaceted beings, comprised of unconscious yet distinctly different parts. They found that while these parts do not have the autonomy of alters in dissociative identity disorder, they are disparate enough from each other that they can be addressed separately in a type of hypnosis they call *ego state therapy*, also known as *parts work*.

In this hypnotic clinical creative trance, previously unconscious aspects of the personality are called separately into dialogue with the conscious mind. Consciously experiencing formerly hidden parts of the self engenders greater awareness and may open a path to an improved psychological integration. Paradoxically, seeing separate parts of the personality creates a greater wholeness. After the parts are acknowledged and difficulties with their functioning are resolved, there can be a new healthy psychological fusion, as the now improved parts meld into a stronger core self.

I use hypnotic ego state therapy with patients, and I am often surprised, as are they, about the parts of the personality that surface and call for attention. This type of clinical creative trance can be very effective in eating disorders where a neglected aspect of the self may be brought forward to establish more healthy food habits and the ability to maintain a desired weight. The parts have the autonomy of their own names, and when they are heard and cared for, they fuse back into the main personality to establish a new healthier phase of living. That the parts emerged fully formed, and capable of dialogue and healing, indicates the vast potential of the unconscious mind.

CHAPTER 4

Empathy and Dissociation in the Creative Trance

Our brains have been designed to blur the line between self and other
Frans de Waal

I have always preferred inspiration to information
Man Ray

Empathy and dissociation, which appear to be opposites, are both intrinsic to the creative trance. Empathy provides the connection between the creative person and the work produced, while dissociation separates the trance state from waking consciousness, and they both exist on a spectrum. Empathy ranges from its presence in everyday relationships, through its centrality in a creative trance, to its highest form as a realization of universal oneness. Dissociation can range from a slight experience of separateness from one's surroundings in daily life, through the cocoon it creates during work in a creative trance, to a loss of individual self-awareness as part of a spiritual experience.

Empathy: The Empathic Trance and Universal Connections

Empathy appears to be its own type of trance state. When we experience empathy, we empathically expand our awareness to intuit the consciousness of another. In this expansion of awareness beyond ourselves, empathy has aspects of an altered state of consciousness. As the ability to see our self in someone else's condition, everyday empathy forms connections and strengthens our bond with human and nonhuman animals. When empathy is a principal factor in the creative trance, it becomes an empathic trance and an altered state of consciousness.

In an empathic trance, the intensity of fusion during the creative process between the creative individual and the work produced, whether it is a painting, a novel, an invention, or a symphony, may form a bond strong

49

enough to rival waking consciousness by obliterating stimuli from the external world. In this way empathy has connections with absorption (Tellegen & Atkinson, 1974). When empathy further extends to realize a connection with the oneness of all being, it evolves beyond trance, becoming a profound experience of consciousness that opens into a sense of universal union. Chinese philosophy (Chang, 1970) describes this metaphysical aspect of empathy, by saying that all distinctions between subject and object disappear. Instead, there is an experience of the Tao, an awareness of the way of the universe.

We are biologically predisposed for empathy through the mirror neuron system in our brain. This assembly of dedicated neurons mirrors the behavior, emotions, and actions of others (Rajmohan & Mohandas, 2007; Pool-Goudzwaard et al., 2018). Orloff (2017) notes that the capacity for empathy in people exists on a spectrum and suggests that individuals high in empathy may have food and caffeine sensitivities along with a tendency to hypoglycemia. Empathy appears related to, yet also paradoxical to the theory of mind. In Theory of Mind, we realize that the emotions, cognition, behavior, and beliefs of another person are different from our own (Şahin et al., 2019). Empathy begins with the acknowledgement of another's differences, but then paradoxically proceeds to meld with the other person in a process of deeper connection and understanding. We understand most fully when we are not ourselves but that which we seek to understand (Root-Bernstein, 1999).

Empathic Projection across Creative Domains

When empathy drives the creative trance, and creative people project themselves into their work, it becomes an empathic trance with similarities across domains. We see a similar use of empathy in visual art and science with the creative processes of the painter Wu Chen (1280–1354) and the geneticist Barbara McClintock (1902–1992), who both empathically projected themselves into their work (Richards & Goslin-Jones, 2018). Wu Chen's paintings of bamboo were considered portraits of the artist as bamboo because he infused himself so completely into their forms. While examining meiosis in the Neurospora fungus, which is its reproductive cell division, McClintock felt she was inside the cells, viewing the interior parts of the chromosomes, and that they were her friends.

Temple Grandin (b. 1947), a professor of animal science who also designs animal handling facilities, is active in the domains of both science and art (Grandin, 1995; Grandin & Johnson, 2005; Zausner,

2016). With a profound empathy for nonhuman animals that she believes comes from having autism, Grandin says, "Autistic people can think the way animals think" (Grandin & Johnson, 2005, p. 6). Using her empathy and knowledge of animal behavior, Grandin designs handling facilities for animals that treat them humanely, incorporating curved tracks that are closer to their natural movements. She also eliminates sharp contrasts of light and dark that may cause the animal to have visual distress.

The Root-Bernsteins (2001) identify empathy as one of the most important tools of a creative mind and note its occurrence across domains. Although they do not call the deep empathic experiences they cite instances of a creative trance, their descriptions are congruent with creative trance phenomenology. They note that the pianist Claudio Arrau (1903–1991), who felt an empathic sense of communion with the composers he played, believed his empathy had unconscious origins. Empathy can also be central to invention. Alexander Graham Bell (1847–1922) felt he became one with the systems he investigated; and Richard Feynman (1918–1988) thought his way inside electronic devices to comprehend their construction.

Empathic Projection in Acting and Sports

One of the most widely known uses of a creative empathic trance is its prevalence as an acting technique. Now fundamental to acting, empathy was not always central to performance. In response to the melodramatic acting practices of the nineteenth century, which resembled individual recitations by actors facing an audience, Constantin Stanislavski developed a more natural empathic style of performing (Clare, 2017; Schonbrun, 2018). Stanislavski's system, requiring actors to empathically relate to and identify with the characters they portray, became the basis for method acting. It produced a revolution in mid-twentieth-century American film and theater with actors including Marlon Brando (1924–2004), James Dean (1931–1955), Julie Harris (1925–2013), and Montgomery Clift (1920–1966) (Hirsch & Bell, 2014).

Audience response, which is their creative trance, increases through an empathic identification with the characters represented. The more the actor is believable, the deeper the audience trance. The dancer and choreographer Isadora Duncan (1877–1927) wanted her performances to instill a kinesthetic empathy in the audience by generating in them a desire for movement (Root-Bernstein, 2001).

Empathy is also part of the creative trance in competitive sports. When an athlete tries to comprehend what an opponent is thinking, that effort to deeply understand the motives and desires of another person is an example of empathy. Lou Brock (b. 1939) of the St, Louis Cardinals, who was inducted into the Baseball Hall of Fame (n.d.), is known as one of the greatest base stealers of all time. When asked about his method of stealing bases, Brock said that he used empathy (cited in Murphy & White, 1995, p. 49). Brock explained, "So you try to make that pitcher your very close buddy by empathizing with all his moves and all his thoughts. You know at one point he has to commit himself, and then he can't go back on it. I have to too, but he has to first, and that makes a big difference."

The Creative Trance and Empathic Intimacy

It is possible that the creative trance, through empathic projection into the work produced and the sustained labor necessary for its generation, is part of the dynamic creating the strong emotional intimacy that some people feel toward their creative works. This may account for the tendency of certain creative individuals to regard their works as their children. As Freud said (1910/1989, p. 81), "There is no doubt that the creative artist feels towards his works like a father," and Barron (1969, p. 18) believed a person's "ideas are his children." Erno Rubik (b. 1944) speaks about his invention, the Rubik Cube, as if it was his child, saying, "I'm very close to the cube," (cited in Alter, 2020, homepage). "The cube was growing up next to me and right now, it's middle-aged, so I know a lot about it."

In visual art, Michelangelo (1475–1564) and Edvard Munch (1863–1944) both regarded their works as their children (Michelangelo, 1963; Gløersen, 1994). After selling a painting, Joseph Mallord William Turner (1775–1851), who hated to part with his work, lamented, "I've lost one of my children this week" (cited in Kent, 1939, n.p., Plate 66). The writer Charles Dickens (1812–1870) even admitted to having a favorite son (1869, p. v). "Like many fond parents," he said, "I have in my heart of hearts, a favorite child, and his name is David Copperfield."

Structure and the Creative Trance: Delineation and Rules

Empathy, a great facilitator of creativity, may manifest through the experience of a creative trance. As a delineated experience, the creative trance can lend structure to the life of a creative person. Within its activities are the rewards of self-expression, and in its delineation, creativity becomes a *time away from time* in daily life. Instead of the responsibilities of everyday living, a creative trance offers opportunities for self-expression. This experience is so rewarding that it becomes a practice of creative self-care that artists look forward to and cherish. As the visual artist Georgia O'Keeffe (1887–1986) stated (cited in Messinger, 1984, p. 58), "Painting is like a thread that runs through all the reasons for all the other things that make one's life."

While the creative trance is an altered state of consciousness, it is not an amorphous state of consciousness. Across domains, there are rules, traditions, and personal preferences that form the scaffolding of a creative trance. Shaped by individual capabilities and relevant social traditions, the creative trance uses the rules of a domain to structure the work produced. Novices learn the rules and assimilate them to become experts who then use the rules unconsciously. In the Japanese tradition (Bowie, 1952), a beginning painter learns different types of brushstrokes to portray diverse aspects of the natural world. Some brushstrokes depict mountains, others are for trees, water, flowers, or people. They form a visual vocabulary that a novice keeps in mind when painting. Yet an experienced artist, having assimilated this visual vocabulary, uses the rules of painting unconsciously, just as a speaker or a writer uses the rules of grammar.

The dynamic of a novice consciously following rules that an expert uses unconsciously is active across domains. Both music and sports start with deliberately learned movements that eventually become unconscious abilities (Kruglanski & Gigerenzer, 2011). While a beginning musician may follow rules with great attention, a professional can follow the same rules without consciously being aware of them. Two experiments in sports, one in golf and the other in soccer, show that consciously thinking about rules guides the work of beginners but can impair the performance of experts (Beilock et al., 2002). When skilled golf players were told to concentrate on the multiple movements inherent in their golf swing, their performance diminished, and when accomplished soccer players were instructed to dribble using their nondominant foot, the concentration required lessened their performance.

Exceptions to this pattern may occur when a skill is not learned by instruction but by observation because then rules are not represented in the form of language (Kruglanski & Gigerenzer, 2011). There is also a difference between rule conforming, which is a rigid adherence to precepts, and rule following, where rules are malleable and can be bent or altered. Malleability is important for creativity. While rules facilitate greater communication through recognized forms and standards of excellence, their flexibility allows for originality. It is assimilating and transcending rules that open the possibilities for originality and excellence.

Structure and the Creative Trance: Preferences and Habitual Behaviors

Another aspect of structure in the creative trance is personal preference, which may manifest as individualized rituals and habitual behaviors that offer a familiar setting and psychological safety to the creative person. Preferences may include arranging supplies in a specific manner, controlling the time needed for creativity, and working in a favorite place. These accustomed and repeated actions can be soothing, enhance security, and allow creativity to emerge. In their calming familiarity and easy repetition, these rituals may become moving meditations of self-care, creating their own trance state, an induction leading into the creative process.

Instilling a sense of calm and control, they open the mind to receptivity and the active surrender of inspiration. Preferences provide a safe foundation of the known that can become a springboard into the creative unknown. Enhancing the experience of flow (Csikszentmihalyi, 1990), personal preferences can promote a state of optimal creativity (Combs & Krippner, 2007), clearing distractions, calming waking awareness, and allowing creative expression to emerge seemingly without effort.

Individualized rituals were important to the self-taught visual artist Grandma Moses (1860–1961). She liked to paint in a sunny room at the east side of her house, working on a table given to her long ago by an aunt (Moses, 1952; Kallir, 1973). With her brushes, paint tubes, and jars of paint laid out in front of her in a specific order, and a board covered with newspapers on the table to protect its surface, Grandma Moses would begin to paint. She filled all her canvases with images from memory. Memory structured her creative trance.

Grandma Moses described it as, "Memory is history recorded in our brain, memory is a painter, it paints pictures of the past and of the day" (Moses, 1952, p. 3). Personal control of time was another fundamental structure of creativity for Grandma Moses. She did not like to be hurried, stating, "I love to take my time and finish things up right" (Moses, 1952, p. 132). Keeping busy was also very important to Grandma Moses, who was an active person, even at an extremely advanced age. Acknowledging that creativity filled and structured her life, she said (Moses, 1952, p. 138), "If I didn't start painting, I would have raised chickens."

Dissociation and Its Definitions

Like empathy, dissociation is an integral part of the creative trance, and encompasses a wide range of experiences. Existing on a spectrum, dissociation can range from feelings of mild detachment from one's surroundings, to sensations of external inspiration, to transcendent experiences with intimations of the divine. The American Psychological Association (2020) gives definitions of dissociative conditions, yet it does not provide a definition for the noun *dissociation*. In response, I will use descriptors offered by Krippner (1997a), who describes dissociation as experiences and actions that appear to be apart from or disconnected from the mainstream of conscious awareness, usual behaviors, and/or an individual's self-identity. As with many conditions, dissociation has both positive and negative aspects, and can no longer be exclusively pathologized. Krippner notes that dissociative experiences may be adaptive or maladaptive, life potentiating or life de-potentiating, and they can be either controlled or uncontrolled.

The Creative Trance and Dissociation

The creative trance encompasses a wide range of dissociative experiences that vary according to the depth of the trance, the personality of the creative person, and the circumstances surrounding the creative work. Dissociation, which may be a negative factor in mental illness (World Health Organization, 1992; American Psychiatric Association, 2013), can be a gateway to inspiration in a creative trance. Like empathy, creative dissociation exists on a spectrum. Starting with brief dissociative experiences that may interrupt waking consciousness with insights and clarifications, it can deepen into the dissociative immersion of inspiration in a creative trance, and further progress to numinous experiences of profound spirituality. Ascending to states beyond trance, dissociation may open into awe and intimations of the ineffable. At all levels, creative dissociation can facilitate a change in consciousness, bringing in new ideas with a transformed view of life.

The maladaptive uncontrolled aspects of dissociation are evident in the clinical pathology of dissociative disorders, where involuntary alterations in identity, consciousness, memory, awareness, and/or motor functions result in impairment and distress (APA, 2020). Negative dissociation can also take the form of dissociative conversion disorders, including dissociative fugue and dissociative stupor, as well as other dissociative disorders, such as dissociative psychosis, dissociative coma, and Ganser syndrome, a dissociative disorder where individuals may mimic mental illnesses (World Health Organization, 1992; American Psychiatric Association, 2013).

When used as an aspect of impaired emotional functioning, dissociation may act as a defense mechanism by keeping away threatening ideas, discomfort with ambiguities, or inner conflicts, through compartmentalizing and separating them away from the main part of the psyche (APA, 2007). Physical conditions that may have uncontrolled dissociation include encephalitis, strokes, sleep disorders, dementia, temporal lobe epilepsy, and a severance of the cerebral commissure between the two hemispheres of the brain, among others (Krippner, 1997a). While these are examples of negative uncontrolled dissociation, the positive controlled dissociation of a creative trance is central to creativity.

Dissociation and Inspiration in the Creative Trance

The creative trance is a dissociative life-potentiating experience, pivotal to the creative process and profoundly different from negative dissociative conditions. As a positive controlled experience, the creative trance is inherently structured by the domain and tradition in which it occurs. Negative uncontrolled dissociation involves fragmentation of the personality and a diminution of consciousness, but the dissociation in a creative trance can cohere and enlarge consciousness through the experience of inspiration.

Dissociative inspiration may feel like a release from the bonds of the ego. Transcending the limits of the ordinary self (Grosso, 1997), inspiration may bring a sense of augmented abilities that seem to come from a source outside of the person or from a previously unreachable part of the mind. Some individuals who believe it originates outside of themselves may call it an inspiration from the Muses, either mythologically (Hamilton, 1969) or through its embodiment in an inspiring personal relationship (Tutter, 2017), while others may experience it as an opening to the divine.

In talks with the musicologist Arthur Abell (1994, p. 117), the composer Giacomo Puccini (1858–1954) insisted the music for his opera *Madame Butterfly* "was dictated to me by God. I was merely instrumental in putting it on paper and communicating it to the public." Then Abell reminded Puccini, "but to do all that, you had to have knowledge and technical skill of a high order." "Of course," replied Puccini, "that is self-understood." Then he said a composer "must acquire by laborious study and application the technical mastery of his craft; but he will never write anything of lasting value unless he has Divine aid also."

The singer, songwriter, and musician Stevie Wonder (Stevland Hardaway Morris, b. 1950) also sees his music as coming from a divine source and says, "I'm only being used as a vehicle" (cited in Rowden, 2012, pp. 115–116). While not every person may believe that their inspiration comes from the divine, examples of creative people experiencing what appears to be an outside source of inspiration occur across domains and cultures (Grosso, 1997). As the poet Percy Bysshe Shelley (1792–1822) stated, "One after another, the greatest writers, poets, and artists confirm the fact that their work comes to them from beyond the threshold of consciousness" (cited in Harmon & Rheingold, 1984, p. 49).

Creativity without Continuous Inspiration

Yet creative people must produce work even though they may not be continually inspired. Inspiration is not constant; it ebbs and flows like the tides but without their predictable regularity. The ocean, a symbol of the unconscious in Jungian psychology (Ronnberg & Martin, 2010), may at high tide bring treasures of inspiration onto the beach of conscious awareness, while at low tide, it seems further away and less accessible. To keep productive, an individual must work in all tides. As the writer E. B. White insisted, "A writer who waits for ideal conditions under which to work will die without putting a word on paper" (cited in Plimpton, 1988).

An important aspect of the creative process is the confidence that work with its creative trance will generate inspiration. The composer Pyotr Ilyich Tchaikovsky (1840–1893) strongly believed that inspiration comes to those who create, insisting that "We must always work, and a self-respecting artist must not fold his hands on the pretext that he is not in the mood . . . We must be patient and believe that inspiration will come" (cited in M. Tchaikovsky, 1906, p. 281). The writer Isabel Allende, who begins all her books on January 8, reiterates this sentiment saying (cited in Moran, 2013, p. 6), "Show up, show up, show up, and after a while the muse shows up, too."

By self-generating a creative trance, work can bring inspiration, although it may still feel like an external gift. In this altered state of consciousness, with its greater opening into the unconscious mind, previously hidden perceptions become more accessible to waking awareness. Taking the form of creative insights, they may seem like gifts from beyond conscious awareness. Yet with them come responsibilities to give in return, because creativity is the transmutation of inspired ideas into shared communication. As the writer Franz Kafka (1883–1924) said (cited in Janouch, 2012, p. 48), "Art like prayer is a hand outstretched in the darkness, seeking for some touch of grace which will transform it into a hand that bestows gifts."

Dissociation and the Elevation of Consciousness

Krippner's (1997a, p. 340) statement that "dissociation once served and continues to serve adaptive functions in human evolution" is evident when dissociation enhances consciousness. Grosso (1997) calls the influence of adaptive dissociation on the elevation of consciousness a *creative dissociation* (p. 193), a state with similarities to the creative trance. He finds creative dissociation to be basic to surrealism, a movement in visual art and literature, influenced by the psychology of Sigmund Freud, that started in Paris during the early 1920s. Grosso believes that surrealism, with its focus on the properties and potential of the unconscious mind, aims to instill an elevation of consciousness by using cognitive dissonance to stimulate a dissociative process that creates distance from ordinary reality.

Cognitive dissonance is basic to surrealists, who engage in automatic writing, find words through Freudian free association, and combine words and images in ways that appear incompatible with the logic of the conscious mind. Surrealist paintings depict dreamscapes, where space-time seems altered with incongruous objects and perspectives, yet their images are painted with vivid clarity to further confuse the distinction between real and unreal. In its efforts to transcend customary waking life, Grosso believes surrealism uses dissociative processes intended to loosen the limitations of the ego and induce a new level of awareness. The surrealists aimed for a dissociative stimulation of consciousness, not only in the artist but also in the viewer, what this book identifies as an audience creative trance.

Dissociative Trance Disorder: A Numinous Cultural Experience

As a positive, controlled, and structured dissociation, trance is not only used in creative expression but also for group cohesion and the transmission of cultural and spiritual values. Trance can be the vehicle that transforms a performance into a numinous event, allowing it to transcend profane individual experience and attain a transtemporal perspective that Mircea Eliade (1975, p. 178) calls "the very source of spiritual existence."

This positive aspect is seen clearly in what the APA (2020) identifies as dissociative trance disorder. Taking care to associate the condition with cultural norms and not to pathologize it, APA describes dissociative trance disorder as containing two subtypes, possession trance and trance disorder, also known as possession trance disorder and trance and possession disorder. During a possession trance the person's identity is replaced by what appears to be an external force such as a divine being or spirit, resulting in loss of memory for the duration of the trance. In trance disorder, individuals keep their identity, but experience altered perceptions of their surroundings.

APA notes these two experiences are customary in the religious practices of various cultures and should not be pathologized unless the cultural or spiritual group considers them to be abnormal. In instances when religious trance possessions are negative, individuals may seek treatment from local healers or denominational clergy. Negative trance states in Indigenous cultures are now being examined as dissociative disorders in contemporary psychology (Ferracuti et al., 1996; van Duijl et al., 2013, 2014).

Dissociation, Ritualized Possession, and the Dance Creative Trance

Worldwide, possession trance and trance disorder are foundations of ritualized creative trance states that keep cultural traditions alive and promote group solidarity. Both types of possession trances may be enhanced by wearing masks and costumes, such as those of the ceremonial story tellers of the Native American Kwakwaka'wakw, living on the Pacific Northwest Coast of North America (Berman, 2000; Cullon, 2013), the dancing monks in the Tibetan tradition (Ricard, 2003), and by ritual dancers of the Chewa and Luvale people in Africa (Phiri, 2008; Nthala, 2011). During ceremonial experiences, the creative trance engendered by the ritual performer becomes a shared creative trance with the audience. In these cases, an audience steeped in the traditions of the performer also judges the authenticity and depth of the performer's trance state.

The anthropologist Grant M. Nthala (2011), who is of Chewa descent, spoke with a man no longer allowed to perform the sacred Chewa ceremonial *gulewamkulu* dance. Despite the former dancer's mask, costume, and ability to dance well, the audience perceived him as being too much himself and not the divine spirit he was supposed to embody. Nthala

(p. 70) quotes the man as saying, "As a result, women easily recognized me when I was in the gulewamkulu gear, and so I was advised by the elders to stop dancing though I was a very good dancer." He had the ability but not the ecstasy, and this was a sacred event. The dancer gave the audience a skillful performance, but they were seeking a numinous experience.

A related but opposite event occurred during a Tamil Hindu ceremony in the East Ham district of London. David (2009) recounts an occasion in the Sri Murugan temple when a devotee in the audience became possessed. As the man danced in trance, other devotees encouraged him by chanting the name of the deity they believed resided within him. Then, identifying the man as an embodiment of the divinity, they offered their children to him for blessings. In the Hindu religion those who are possessed and embodying a deity are regarded as divine for the length of their possession. It is an emotionally healing and numinous experience for the possessed and for the other devotees. In profound spiritual experiences, the creative trance can lead to transcendence, which is a state beyond trance. As David (2009, p. 222) says, for these participants, there is a "taste of the divine, or being absorbed in a greater sense of self which brings enjoyment and peace as a fully emotional and transcendent experience."

Coincidentia Oppositorum: The Paradoxical Union of Empathy and Dissociation

The devotee in the temple is simultaneously in a dissociative and an empathic state, being separated from his normal waking consciousness and merged with a deity. Here, dissociation and empathy combine, leading to an ecstasy of transcendence. The word *ecstasy*, as Combs (2002, p. 342) points out, derives from the Greek *stasis*, to stand, and *ex*, as outside, which combine to mean outside of our ordinary mind. He then notes that in transcendent states such as samadhi, consciousness usually turns inward, and suggests using the word *entasy*, coming from the Greek, *en* for inside and *stasis* to stand. Yet it is possible that both words apply to the states of transcendence that open up from the deepest depths of a human being to the highest reaches of the creative trance.

These experiences appear to derive from the opposite natures of empathy and dissociation that create a paradoxical union in the creative trance and the states beyond it. Ecstasy would be the dissociation from ordinary awareness, while entasy would be an empathic inner union with the divine. In their simultaneous occurrence and their fusion, they create both a paradox and pinnacle of human consciousness. The end of their dichotomy is the nature of their paradox. Through their unification of opposites, they are a *coincidentia oppositorum*, with interpenetration and interdependence (Drob, 2000) creating a profound mystical experience. In analytical psychology (Jung, 1977), a resolution of opposites is mediated by the transcendent function, indicating an inner transformation on the path to individuation and realization.

CHAPTER 5

Evolution, Altered States, and the Creative Trance

Upper Paleolithic people must have experienced not only "normal con-sciousness" but also altered consciousness because altered states are wired into the human nervous system

David Lewis-Williams & Jean Clottes

Art is universal because each human was designed by evolution to be an artist

John Tooby & Leda Cosmides

We are creative primates who evolved from creative primates, and as our cognition increased so did the complexity of our creative trance. In the evolutionary history of our symbolic communication, even early works suggest altered states and transformation of the self. There are archaic artifacts with symbols that intimate initiation and life after death, prehis-toric images on cave walls intended to influence both affect and reality, and talismanic objects linked to altered states, rituals, and healing. Our tool-making that evolved from everyday objects advanced to devices that could alter civilizations, expanding human cognitive capacity with external memory devices like alphabets, computers, and the digital cloud.

The Earliest Hominin Tools: Lomekwian Stone Tools from Kenya

A hallmark of hominin creativity is constructing and using tools. Currently, primates such as orangutans, chimpanzees, and capuchin mon-keys all use tools in the wild (Bird & Emery, 2009), and it is likely that our pre-hominin primate ancestors used them as well. The earliest tools were simple and utilitarian, but eventually they became more complex, incorp-orating aesthetic considerations and greatly increasing the number of variables, generating a multifaceted creative trance. While it is not possible to say this with certainty because behavior does not fossilize (Tooby & Cosmides, 2005), the evidence remains in their creative products.

Currently, the earliest examples of toolmaking in the history of human evolution are the 3.3 million BP (before present) Lomekwian stone tools from West Turkana in Kenya (Harmand et al., 2015). Yet they were discovered by accident (Balter, 2015). When Harmand and her colleagues were in West Turkana looking for evidence of an ancient hominin, Kenyanthropus platyops, they made a wrong turn in their search and found themselves in an area called Lomekwi. There, exposed on the surface of a slope deposit, were stones that they recognized as ancient artifacts and immediately started an excavation. In this classic example of the creative trance of discovery, past knowledge and experience use current stimuli for an inspired breakthrough. As Pasteur famously noted, chance favors the prepared mind (Pearce, 1912).

It is not certain which early species created the more than one hundred tools found at the archaeological site. Dating from the Pliocene, they are before the emergence of our genus Homo and may possibly be the work of Kenyanthropus platyops or Australopithecus afarensis (Harmand et al., 2015). The Lomekwian artifacts are large pieces of knapped rock, which means they are stones struck by other stones so that pieces flake off to create a sharp edge usable for cutting, scraping, and chopping (Lombard et al., 2019).

Oldowan Stone Tools from Tanzania: The River-Worn Cobble and Possible Aesthetics

A further step in tool evolution are the smaller, smoother Oldowan stone tools, dating from the 2.6 million BP Lower Paleolithic, found in Tanzania's Olduvai Gorge (Harmand et al., 2015). Their craftsmanship and the hominin remains discovered near the site by Mary and Louis Leakey led Leakey and his colleagues (Leakey et al., 1964, p. 8) to propose a new species, *Homo habilis*, meaning Handyman, someone who is able and mentally skillful. The Oldowan knapped tools, which have been attributed to the creativity of Homo habilis (Donald, 1991; Gabora & Kaufman, 2010), may possibly be the work of other early hominins (Susman, 1991; De Heinzelin et al., 1999).

Lighter, smoother, and more graceful than the rough-edged Lomekwian artifacts, the Oldowan tools may have been the result of a creative inspiration to use a large river-worn pebble or cobble as a core stone to be knapped instead of an irregular piece of rock. Possibly this type of creative trance occurred multiple times to different individuals. By holding a core stone in one hand and striking it with a harder stone used as a hammerstone/chisel they constructed a usable cutting edge. This free-hand percussion method (Harmand et al., 2015) offered more control over the size and position of the detaching flake.

Unlike the early Lomekwian tools, which appear to be strictly utilitarian, the later Oldowan tools suggest the beginning of aesthetic decisions and by inference a more nuanced creative trance. Although some Oldowan tools are made of plain stone, others are crafted in green lava, which Pfeiffer (1982) cites as an aesthetic choice. Harrod (2014b, p. 135) proposes that seven Oldowan plain stone artifacts, including a "grooved and pecked cobble" from approximately 1.8 million BP, exhibit possible nonutilitarian aesthetic modifications.

The Acheulean Handaxe: Aesthetic Choices, Increased Craftsmanship, and Works of Art

In the Lower Paleolithic, at about 1.8 million BP with the arrival of Homo erectus, human evolution brought more definitive aesthetic decisions, a higher level of craftsmanship, and an increasingly complex creative trance. Originally from Africa, Homo erectus eventually migrated throughout the Indian subcontinent and Europe (Donald, 1991, 1995, 2006; Lycett, 2009). Adapting to many different climates, and living in societies with cooperation and coordinated action, Homo erectus created the Acheulean handaxe.

This bilaterally knapped stone tool, with its flake-flattened front and back surfaces, was sculpted into a symmetrical oval, triangular, or teardrop shape with a sharp cutting edge (Pfeiffer, 1982; Lycett, 2009). Requiring from twenty-five up to sixty-five strikes to carve, it first appeared about 1.7 million to 1.6 million BP. By 500,000 BP, the handaxes were accompanying hominin migration to the Near East, Europe, and the Indian subcontinent.

Acheulean handaxes vary in their degree of craftsmanship and aesthetics. Some are plain stones, but others feature embedded fossils prominently centered in the tool as an obvious aesthetic decision. A handaxe discovered in Norfolk, UK, displays a fossil shell of the mollusk *Spondylus spinosus* while another handaxe from Kent, UK, features a fossil of the echinoid *Conulus* (Pfeiffer, 1982; Dissanayake, 1988). These tools, carefully sculpted to feature the fossil as a precious jewel, are objects of beauty. By attaining the level of art, they may be the oldest works of purposeful art in the hominin line. These carefully produced handaxes, which were made by Homo erectus, infer that the creation of visual art predates the rise of modern humans.

The Acheulean Handaxe: Early Hominins and Symbolic Communication

Intentionally aesthetic, these handaxes might not have been used for everyday tasks, but possibly created as social, hierarchical, or ceremonial objects of value. Kohn and Mithen (1999) believe that their attractive symmetry may have been used as a social display to attract a mate. Creating objects with considerable forethought, planning, artistic skill, and possibly symbolic thought indicates the presence of a more complex creative trance. In response, the final product elicits what Dissanayake (1988, p. 95) identifies as "aesthetic satisfaction," inspiring an audience trance of appreciation in the viewer and user. As an art-making species that evolved from art-making species, symbolic behavior also appears to be part of our heritage.

Acheulean handaxes, which take considerable ability to construct, also require social skills to transmit the information about their manufacture and use. Presumably lacking the anatomy for modern speech (Lieberman, 2007), Donald (1995) believes that Homo erectus may have communicated in a concrete situation-bound symbolic manner through gesture, sound, body language, event-reenactment, pantomime, and expressive group behavior. He describes this as a mimetic culture, deriving from the word *mime*, and sees it as a forerunner to modern syntactic language. It is possible that in these mimetic behaviors that transmit information, we can see the archaic origins of modern acting, mime, performance art, theater, choral expression, and audience appreciation.

Figurative Art in the Lower Paleolithic: Carved Likenesses in the Art of Hominins

Thoughts of prehistoric figurative art usually recall works from the Upper Paleolithic, such as the 12,000–17,000 BP paintings on the cave walls at Lascaux, Niaux, and Altamira, near the Pyrenees (Valladas et al., 2001), or the c. 25,000 BP Venus of Willendorf sculpture (Antl-Weiser, 2009). Yet recent research has found much earlier works, two small figurines from the

Lower Paleolithic: the Berekhat Ram and the Tan-Tan. These two carvings, sometimes called *Venuses*, are the earliest examples of single female figurines, a type of sculpture found throughout the Upper Paleolithic.

Initially there were concerns that the figurines were manuports, which are unmodified natural objects that have been carried away from their place of origin like the Makapansgat cobble. This very unusual 8.3-millimeter-high piece of jasperite rock dating from the Pliocene at 2.5 to 3 million BP has two hominin faces, one on each side, although there is no evidence of any anthropic alteration (Dart, 1974; Bednarik, 1998).

Unlike the Makapansgat cobble, microscopic research indicates that the two figurines were intentionally carved (Marshack, 1997; d'Errico & Nowell, 2000; Bednarik, 2003). For both sculptures, a naturally occurring small piece of rock was altered by incising lines to increase its resemblance to a hominin form. Here, the creative trance would begin with a type of pattern recognition. Called visual ambiguity, it is the capacity to recognize the familiar in an ambiguous form (Flounders et al., 2019), such as seeing the possibility of an anthropomorphic shape in the yet unaltered stone. We are biologically prone to visual ambiguity, from its use in detecting threats to its centrality in facial recognition and bonding. With pattern recognition as inspiration, the creative trance might continue with successive visualizations of the incisions needed to alter the stones to a more identifiable figurative form.

Lower Paleolithic Figurines: The Berekhat Ram and the Tan-Tan

The first figurine found was the Berekhat Ram. Dating from approximately 250,000 to 280,000 BP, it was unearthed in the Golan Heights in Israel (Goren-Inbar, 1986; Marshack, 1997; d'Errico et al., 2003). The great age of the figurine puts it well before the appearance of modern humans, making it more contemporaneous with the Acheulean culture (Goren-Inbar, 1986), and possibly attributable to Homo heidelbergensis (Morriss-Kay, 2010). Made of basaltic lapillus tuff with scoria clasts, which is a type of dark basalt volcanic rock, the Berekhat Ram is the size of a pebble, measuring only 1.38 inches (3.5 cm) in height.

The naturally rounded form of the rock appears to be intentionally incised with several lines to increase its resemblance to the female body (Marshack, 1997; d'Errico & Nowell, 2000). With what appear to be large breasts and an extended middle part of the figure, the Berekhat Ram is suggestive of a pregnant female hominin. It may have been used symbolically as a fertility totem, a talismanic object to elicit an altered state in the viewer.

Fertility would have been very important to Paleolithic hominins, where every birth was crucial to the survival of their small communities.

An even earlier stone figurine, the Tan-Tan, was found in the banks of the River Draa, just south of the town of Tan-Tan in Morocco (Bednarik, 2003). Dating from 300,000 to 500,000 BP and made of metamorphosed quartzite, it measures 2.29 inches (58.2 mm) high. Like the Berekhat Ram, it is an anthropomorphically shaped rock, altered to increase its resemblance to a hominin form. The Tan-Tan may possibly be the work of Homo heidelbergensis (Morriss-Kay, 2010). Five out of its eight grooves appear to be intentionally incised, and traces of ochre found on the figurine strongly suggest its use as a ritual object. The ochre's reddish coloring would intensify the figurine's lifelike resemblance and serve to increase its perception as an object of power. Using totems in a ritual can deepen the altered states of participants, and Vernon (2019) believes that shared trance states, such as those in religious and spiritual traditions, have been central to cultural evolution.

Homo Sapiens and the Modern Creative Trance: Artifacts from Blombos Cave

Fossil evidence suggests that modern human beings, Homo sapiens, first appeared in Africa approximately 300,000 BP (Gibbons, 2017) with a corresponding increase in creativity there that spread to the Near East with successive waves of migration (d'Errico et al., 2003). Some of the earliest examples of Homo sapien creativity are the Middle Stone Age artifacts found in Blombos Cave, at Southern Cape in South Africa (d'Errico et al., 2001; Henshilwood et al., 2002, 2009, 2018). The African Middle Stone Age is approximately equal to the Middle Paleolithic (Henshilwood & Sealy, 1997).

The Blombos Cave artifacts include two pieces of incised ochre dating from 75,000 BP, thirteen pieces of incised ochre dating from 75,000 to 100,000 BP, an engraved bone fragment from 70,000 BP, and what is currently the oldest known rock drawing from 73,000 BP. All the objects exhibit an intentionally created pattern, with some showing a crosshatched design. While the ochre and bone pieces are incised with patterns, the design on the rock fragment was painted using liquid ochre.

Homo Sapiens and the Modern Creative Trance: Symbolism and Suggestions of Ritual

The patterned pieces of Middle Stone Age art exemplify what Dissanayake (1992, p. 42) calls "making special," the enhancement of a raw object into a decorated one (Lévi-Strauss, 1970). While the intentional patternings on these objects are aesthetic decisions with possible symbolic or spiritual meanings, the similarity of some of their designs suggests the expression of a cultural tradition (d'Errico et al., 2001; Henshilwood & d'Errico, 2011). On at least one of the incised ochre pieces, the crosshatched set of markings is placed within borders that conform to the edge of the piece. This creates a frame for the markings, showing further intentionality, and presenting it as a planned geometric design.

Boas (1955) believes that in primitive artifacts, abstract geometric forms may encode an important meaning for the society that created them. The presence of meaning and symbolism in the ochres infer their possible use in religious or shamanic ceremonies (Henshilwood, 2009) where they might be considered sacred objects, generating a profound response in a viewer aware of their symbolism. Symbolic thinking creates a cascade of thoughts, linked inner associations that arise and can deeply influence an altered state during rituals. Social traditions also shape an artist's creative trance because the person is a conduit for the culture.

A Middle Stone Age Art Workshop at Blombos Cave

In addition to the carved pieces of ochre discovered at Blombos Cave, over eight thousand pieces of plain ochre were found there (Henshilwood, 2009), along with evidence of the oldest known art workshop (Henshilwood et al., 2011). In this ochre-processing art workshop from 100,000 BP, the liquid ochre mixture was made and kept in two abalone shells (Haliotis midae). Their nacreous pearlescent inner surfaces may have also served as a palette to see the colors more clearly. Ochres, which are mineralized colored earths, are still in use today as pigments and these mixes may be the first art supplies found in a workshop setting. Citing evidence of the conceptual capacity to find, store, and combine substances, using social interactions and the technology of its day, Henshilwood and colleagues (2011, p. 219) believe that Blombos Cave "represents a benchmark in the evolution of complex human cognition."

The contents of the abalone shells suggest meaningful choices and symbolic behavior because their residues show both a yellow-orange ochre pigment and a red ochre pigment, which may have been used for different purposes. Hovers and colleagues (2003) found differently colored ochre pigments in the 92,000 BP Qafzeh cave site south of Nazareth in Israel and believe the ability to separate and choose between them infers evidence of color symbolism. The colored ochres at Blombos Cave may have had specific meanings and uses as well. Contents of a toolkit excavated there included hammerstones, grindstones, bones, and charcoal. It is possible that the charcoal, which makes black marks, was also used for symbolic purposes.

The Blombos Cave workshop appears to be a very early example of a long tradition. Workshops, where art lessons included grinding pigments such as ochres to make paints, played an important part in training artists throughout history. They were central to High Renaissance culture in Italy (Hartt, 1987) and educated Leonardo da Vinci, Michelangelo, Titian, Raphael, and countless other artists. Based on the oral transmission of information from expert to novice along with physical demonstrations of technique, the workshop tradition is a natural way for humans to learn (Zausner, 2016). As a vehicle for the continuation of culture, their guidance shapes the artist's creative trance.

Paleolithic Shell Beads and Their Symbolism

Other examples of meaningful artifacts from Blombos Cave are the 75,000 BP beads made from the shell of the marine gastropod *Nassarius kraussianus* (Henshilwood et al., 2004). Once strung and worn, these perforated snail shells still have traces of ochre. Beads, which are a personal adornment associated with modern human behavior and cognitive abilities, are also symbolic objects (Henshilwood, 2009). In addition to imparting information such as social status and tribal identification, beads may also symbolize spiritual or shamanic power in certain societies. They make the wearer "special" (Dissanayake 1992, p. 42), differentiated from a non-adorned human being, and as impressive objects are meant to elicit a response of admiration in the viewer. Perforating the shells, painting them with ochre, and stringing them add to their "specialness," and would be part of an artist's creative trance during their time of production.

Shell beads, which are still worn today, have been found in multiple and widely dispersed Paleolithic sites, including Algeria, Kenya, Tanzania, Turkey, and Australia (Balme & Morse, 2006). The pierced *Nassarius* shells from Skhul cave in Israel are currently the oldest at 100 to 135,000 BP (Vanhaeren et al., 2006; Bar-Yosef Mayer et al., 2009), and those at Qafzeh are 92,000 BP (Vandermeersch, 2002; d'Errico et al., 2003). Hard, beautiful, with an intricate shape, and a glossy surface, shell beads were the diamonds of their day. They appear to be highly valued, because they were often brought from seashores far away from the sites where they were found (Balme & Morse, 2006; Bar-Yosef Mayer et al., 2009). Their transport suggests trading activity and the possibility of some form of oral language (d'Errico et al., 2001; Henshilwood, 2009).

Shells and the Symbolism of Everlasting Life

Widespread and enduring, the interest in shells extends beyond their physical beauty. Shells appear to have a metaphysical symbolism suggesting altered states and the eternal. Like shorelines and beaches, we are etched by the tides of life, yet intact shells show no such wear. Sparkling and pristine in a seemingly perpetual newness, shells infer immortality by surviving the animals that made them. By outliving the creatures that inhabit them, shells also symbolize the body cast off by the soul at death (De Vries, 1984; Chevalier & Gheerbrant, 1996).

Shells relate to the water where they are found. In Indigenous African religions, water is sacred, and bodies of water are the home of spirits (Ogungbile, 1997). Signifying the spiritual domain in the depth of waters, shells symbolize a safe journey home to the spirits with the promise of immortality in an everlasting life after death (Kozicz, 2017). People in Africa and of African descent in the United States continue this symbolism through their tradition of placing shells on graves (Jamieson, 1995).

With a symbolic association to both death and everlasting life, it is not surprising that shell beads have been excavated at Paleolithic burial sites (d'Errico et al., 2003) such as Skhul cave (Bar-Yosef Mayer et al., 2009). Neanderthals also created and wore a variety of personal decorative ornaments (Henshilwood et al., 2009) and used ochre pigments, suggesting that they, as well as Homo sapiens, may have possessed the capacities for symbolic thought (Hovers et al., 2003; Langley et al., 2008).

Engraved Ostrich Eggshells and Egg Symbolism

At the Diepkloof shelter, a Paleolithic site in South Africa near the Blombos Cave, excavations have uncovered engraved ostrich eggshells from c. 60,000 BP (Henshilwood et al., 2009; Texier et al., 2010). Ostrich eggshells, which carry approximately one liter of water, are used as containers today by contemporary African hunter gatherers and may have served that function in the Middle Stone Age. Yet the engraved eggshells also suggest a possible symbolic and ritual purpose because the egg is an archetypal symbol (ARAS, 2020). Analytical psychology differentiates a local symbol known only to a specific group of people from an archetypal symbol, such as an egg, which has a similarity of meaning across cultures and time (Jung, 1969).

In many traditions around the world from antiquity to the present day, eggs are a symbol of renewal and rebirth (Chevalier & Gheerbrant, 1996). The egg symbolizing a new world is found in the mythology of Japan, Hawaii, Persia, Phoenicia, and India (Von Franz, 1978; Bayley, 1988). Cross-culturally, their symbolism of cosmic renewal is also associated with the symbolic rebirth of an individual (Eliade, 1965, 1975). As an archetypal symbol, it is possible that the people who incised and used the ostrich eggs may have employed them in rituals of rebirth, such as initiation rites, where trance states can be integral to transformation. The ancient initiatory association of the egg most likely originates in the "twofold birth of birds" (Eliade, 1965, p. 54), once as an egg from its mother and again as a chick from its egg.

The egg would symbolize an initiate, who is born once from a maternal womb as a child and then reborn through a rite of initiation to a higher level of wisdom as an adult. The concept of a twice-born human being is a tenet of religious traditions worldwide and central to Indigenous societies where adulthood is achieved through an initiatory rebirth. Initiation reflects our capacity for growth and change. We are evolutionary beings, evolving through both physical evolution and psychological self-evolution with successive initiatory altered states.

Two Paleolithic Stone Artifacts: Incised Flint Plaquettes

Further intimations of initiation rites come from two Paleolithic flint plaquettes. Each plaquette is a stone cortex, a rock with incised lines on the surface of its flat outer layer. The patterned incisions, which are acknowledged to be anthropically created and symbolic (d'Errico et al., 2003), indicate that Middle Paleolithic hominins were able to think symbolically (Hovers et al., 1996). It is not yet known whether the hominin creators of these cortices were Neandertals or anatomically modern human beings (d'Errico et al., 2003). The flint for the cortices is not native to the area where they were found but was transported from ten to twelve kilometers away (Hovers et al., 1996), suggesting it was a valued material.

The first cortex is from Qafzeh cave, south of Nazareth in Israel (Hovers et al., 1996; d'Errico et al., 2003; Hovers, 2009). Dating from 90,000 BP to 100,000 BP, it measures 6.2 w x 4.0 h x 1.6 d cm. The second cortex, dating from c. 54,000 BP and 7.2 cm wide, is incised with similar markings and was discovered in the nearby site of Quneitra (Marshack, 1996). The cortices are thought to be nonutilitarian socially symbolic objects (Hovers et al., 1996), created for a specific, perhaps ritual purpose in the lives of the community (Marshack, 1996).

Both pieces of stone have been deliberately marked with a similar pattern, although the Qafzeh cortex has been broken and only the bottom part of the design remains visible. The similarity of their markings over thousands of years suggests the presence of a continued tradition. There is possible evidence for this tradition extending to the Mousterian levels in Italy, where several incised flint cortices, the size of the Israeli artifacts or slightly larger, were found with a comparable engraved pattern (Hovers et al., 1996). Similar incisions occurring multiple times over an extended geographic area suggest a widespread practice and the importance of the engraved information. Hovers (2009, p. 309) calls incised items "information-encoding devices" and we can presume that similar markings may encode analogous messages.

The Symbolism of the Paleolithic Plaquettes

The incisions on the Qafzeh and Quneitra cortices show semicircular concentric lines surrounding a blank semicircle of clear unaltered stone at the bottom of the plaquette. While some investigations have not found a meaning in the pattern (d'Errico et al., 2003; Morriss-Kay, 2010), others believe it may illustrate a valley (Harrod, 2014b) or a rainbow (Marshack, 1996). In examining the Quneitra cortex, Harrod (2014b) points out that the concentric circular incisions are framed by straight lines forming a triangle shape above them. These lines are only partly visible on the Qafzeh cortex because breakage has cropped the image.

Harrod (2014b), who sees the triangular shape as symbolizing the female vulva, believes the markings show a birthing source. He connects the image with the depiction of a valley and the fertility goddess worship suggested by Paleolithic female figurines. I agree that the image symbolizes a birth, yet not of a child, but the ritualized initiatory rebirth of an individual. An infant being born would require just one circle depicting its head. Yet here there is a semicircular shape at the bottom of the artifact surrounded by multiple arcing semicircular lines radiating out around it. This design suggests an image of a shining sun appearing over the horizon. The rising sun as the coming of light and a new day represents the birth of a new consciousness and a new life, which is a cross-cultural initiatory goal. It is the dawn of a new day symbolizing the dawn of a new life.

Marshack (1996) believes the cortex is a religious symbolic object that would be shown at the culmination of a ceremony. This is when sacred objects are shown to individuals in an altered state who have successfully completed an initiation. It is a time when symbolism would produce a heightened response and the symbols on the cortices appear to be archetypal. Across cultures, the womb is symbolic of the Great Mother, who is the Generatrix of new life (Eliade, 1965), and the sun is a cross-cultural symbol of power and heroism (Cirlot, 1971; Moon, 1991). Both are aspects of an initiation with its goal of rebirth to a higher level of functioning. As archetypal symbols, they are primordial images in the collective unconscious, (Jung, 1973) and according to Jung (1966, pp. 81–82), "Whoever speaks in primordial images speaks with a thousand voices."

Upper Paleolithic Art on the Walls of Caves: Skill and Depth of Meaning

Later migrations out of Africa at approximately 50,000 BP incited an explosion of creative behavior (Klein, 1995; Hovers et al., 2003). In the Franco-Cantabrian area of Upper Paleolithic Europe from about 35,000 to 10,000 BP, it was the time of exquisitely rendered cave art, both painted and engraved (Lewis-Williams & Clottes, 1998; Valladas et al., 2001; Bednarik, 2010; Clottes, 2016). Also known as parietal art, it ranges from cupules, which are small anthropically created cup-shaped depressions in rock, to abstract designs, and realistic depictions of animals, such as those in the *Hall of the Bulls* at Lascaux from 17,000 BP and the bison at Altamira from 15,000 BP. The earliest-known realistic images are on the walls of the Chauvet cave in France, and are radiocarbon dated to more than 30,000 BP (Appenzeller, 1998; Valladas et al., 2001). Many cave art depictions are of animals and appear to be hunting scenes, most likely because accessing sufficient food was crucial to survival for the small bands of Upper Paleolithic humans.

The engravings and images on cave walls may have functioned as visual prayers, hoping to ensure a continued availability of the animals represented. Using art in this way makes it a form of sympathetic magic (Clottes, 2016), where like attracts like. Clottes (2016, p. 10), who notes the presence of hunting scenes to obtain food and images of pregnant animals to continue the food supply, calls it utilitarian magic because the images "were created to influence reality through its representation." The images also appear to be generated to strongly influence an audience creative trance.

Upper Paleolithic Cave Art: Imagery and Altered States

Through their viewing, the animals represented may have been intended to stimulate a psychological or nonmaterial connection between hunter and prey. This altered state of identity-blurring by assuming the mentality of a nonhuman animal is a type of creative trance currently practiced by Australian Aborigine trackers (Sevilla, 2019) and by the San hunters of the Kalahari in South Africa (Guenther, 2017). As one of the San hunters said (p. 3), "You have taken the kudu into your mind." The talismanic images of animals in the caves might have been psychological facilitators for this type of connection. In addition, the images may have functioned as a visual aid to positive psychology. By seeing multiple animals on the cave walls, Paleolithic viewers may have been persuaded that an abundance of animals existed and awaited capture, increasing their optimism and energy for obtaining a food source.

The degree of realism in some of the images intimates the skill to create them was learned and repeatedly honed. It is probable that early humans decorated their homes and more accessible outer caves, but this aspect of their art has been lost in the intervening millennia. While human habitation in the outer caves would have produced continued wear on the painted surfaces of the stone walls, it appears that the absence of imagery may also have been caused by biocorrosion from roosting bats. In their study of bat habitation in the Azé Prehistoric cave, located in Saône-et-Loire, France, Barriquand and associates (2021) find that bat guano deposits form aerosols and acidic leachates that can completely obliterate wall art and damage archaeological artifacts.

Now we are left with only the art of the deep caves, which we are fortunate to have found. The impact of viewing this relatively inaccessible art may intensify an audience creative trance because the works, hidden in caves, make them function as treasures when discovered and seen. Clottes (2016) believes these deep caves were not visited frequently and possibly only by the initiated.

Upper Paleolithic Cave Art: Trance, Shamanism, and the Underworld

Lewis-Williams and Clottes (1998) suggest the decorated caves were places of ritualized altered states. Citing (pp. 14–15) a "neurological bridge" or neuronal similarity between humans of today and those in the Upper Paleolithic, they say Upper Paleolithic people experienced altered states of consciousness because trance states "are wired into the human nervous system." Referring to the three-tiered shamanic cosmology of the upper-world, the middleworld of daily life, and the underworld, they believe that for Upper Paleolithic people, the caves functioned as the underworld and dwelling place of spirits (Clottes & Lewis-Williams, 1998). Here, art and ritualized shamanic trances might serve to function as gateways of contact to a nonmaterial realm.

Across nations, shamanism has been an integral aspect of the spiritual life in hunter-gatherer societies, and it appears to be an active part of Upper Paleolithic culture (Winkelman, 2002). Here intimations of shamanic trance states on the cave walls show certain shaman figures as only partly human, suggesting they have already assumed the form of their spirit animal (Clottes & Lewis-Williams, 1998). There are also geometric abstract designs on the walls, such as patterns of dots, lines, or zigzags that may represent entoptic phenomena. Also known as phosphenes, they are internally produced visual experiences originating from within the brain and the eye.

As interior imagery, these patterns may suggest the first stages of trance, and in some cases might have been augmented through the ingestion of psychotropic substances (Clottes & Lewis-Williams, 1998; Lewis-Williams & Clottes, 1998). Kedar and associates (2021) find that the reduced oxygen content in deep interior caves could cause altered states of consciousness and believe the sites were chosen for that purpose. They note that hypoxia can increase dopamine levels in the brain and may bring sensations of out-of-body experiences and induce hallucinations.

Upper Paleolithic Cave Art: Stone Irregularities, Object Recognition, and Imagery

The placement of cave art further increases its power. When the protrusions, ridges, or cracks in the cave walls suggest an eye or the line of an animal's body, an artist would use the stone's irregularity to create a corresponding image (Hodgson & Pettitt, 2018). This integral connection between stone surface and image may have increased the impact of the art by creating a sense that the animals were manifesting from the underworld through the walls. Thousands of years later, in an example of a similar creative trance, Leonardo da Vinci (1970a) advises artists to stare at stains on a wall and watch them morph into subject matter for paintings.

Seeing an animal or other known entity in the irregularities of a wall is a natural human ability. Called *core object recognition* (DiCarlo et al., 2012,

p. 415), and similar to visual ambiguity, it is the capacity to quickly recognize an object despite considerable variations in its appearance. Occurring through a cascade of brain computations, the recognition culminates as a neuronal pattern in our inferior temporal cortex. This neurological response may be psychologically augmented because as humans we tend to see in schemas projecting the familiar onto the unknown.

Upper Paleolithic Sculpture: The Venus of Willendorf

In addition to stationary parietal art, there are also mobiliary or portable Upper Paleolithic works, such as the small female figurines called *Venuses* found throughout Eurasia. Perhaps the most famous of these is the Venus of Willendorf. Dating from approximately 25,000 BP, this carefully carved oolitic limestone statuette measuring 4.375 inches (11.1 cm) high was found in 1908 near Willendorf, Austria, when excavations for a railroad exposed seven Paleolithic layers (Antl-Weiser, 2009). Although the Venus of Willendorf suggests fertility with her large midsection, full breasts, and prominently displayed genitals (Colman, 1998), it is her obesity (Seshadri, 2012) that surprises modern viewers in an age when tall thin fashion models are the current beauty ideal.

In his examination of multiple Paleolithic female figurines, Józsa (2011) found that fifty-one percent of them depicted an overweight or obese female, leading him to conclude that in the Paleolithic, obesity was the ideal body. This shape would have been as difficult to achieve then as the form of a tall thin fashion model is today. Fertility, which is associated with adequate body weight, would be hard to maintain during the frequent famines and extensive glaciation of Paleolithic Europe (Colman, 1998; Dixson & Dixson, 2011). Undernutrition was a widespread problem at that time, and short lifespans were further attenuated by the high mortality rates of pregnancy and childbirth. In response, Colman (1998, p. 58) suggests that "the Venus of Willendorf may have been used as a talisman in a precarious world of heightened obstetric-related mortality."

The Venus of Willendorf: A Talismanic Figurine

Talismans are meant to produce a very strong audience creative trance in the viewer/recipient. The talismanic aspect of the Venus of Willendorf is intensified by the cap or hair that covers her inclined head and face. Faceless, she is no longer a specific person, but intimates a universal feminine. With her shrouded head tilted downward, she suggests the interior focus of a figure in trance, adding to her power as a totem. Arms and hands are a sign of strength but the Venus of Willendorf has very thin underrepresented arms and hands, so they are not her strength. Her power appears to be in her strongly represented breasts, midsection, and genitals, suggesting she may be the talisman of a fertility goddess. Her feet, which have partly broken, are too small to balance the body, indicating the figurine was probably meant to be a handheld totem. Traces of reddish ochre further infer ritualistic use by making the statuette "special" (Dissanayake, 1992, p. 42) and more lifelike.

As a possible obstetric/fertility totem, the Venus of Willendorf might have been used to lessen discomfort during labor and childbirth. Talismans, revered as objects of power, may induce altered states with analgesic placebo effects that reduce the sensation of pain. Called placebo analgesia, it is a neurobiological response to psychological factors (Zion & Crum, 2018). These factors include mindset, anticipation, and the power of suggestion, as well as psychosocial forces in the environment, such as a community's belief in the efficacy of the totem. Evolutionarily adaptive (Thompson et al., 2009), the placebo effect may work by releasing the body's endogenous opioids and may include a release of dopamine in the basal ganglia because of dopamine's role in associating stimulus with reward (Oken, 2008). Placebo analgesia also appears to reduce the experience of pain by decreasing brain activity in regions that process pain, such as the thalamus, the insula, and the anterior cingulate cortex (ACC), while being strongly correlated with an enhanced amplitude of alpha waves (De Pascalis et al., 2021).

Spirituality appears to strengthen the placebo experience (Kohls et al., 2011), and it is presumed the Venus of Willendorf was administered ritualistically. Another possible source of placebo generation may stem from the figurine's archetypal nature as a comforting nurturing facet of the Great Mother (Neumann, 1974). In this soothing aspect, it also might have been used to reduce experiences of non-obstetric pain. The placebo response, as an audience creative trance, could be intensified by the intimacy of a handheld object. In certain altered states where the impossible may seem attainable, how much more attainable might the impossible seem if you were holding it in your hand.

Evolving Creative Achievements across Domains and Social Responsibility

The Middle to Upper Paleolithic era was a time of extraordinary creativity (Gabora & Kaufman, 2010; Gabora & DiPaola, 2012). Humans made musical instruments, decorated pottery, and left indications of dance. It was also a time of ornate burial sites, signifying the presence of religion, ritual, and metaphysical beliefs. Capable of fluid thinking between divergent and convergent thought processes, along with symbolic reasoning, humans would eventually create stories with metaphors and analogies (Donald, 1991; Gabora & Kaufman, 2010). With sophisticated communication came metacognition and its ability for reflection and self-awareness. These advanced capacities combined with the creation of complex works of art gave rise to the existence of the modern creative trance.

Addressing the question of why humans are creative, Gabora and Kaufman (2010) believe that creativity is both compelling and driven by evolutionary forces. Comparing the drive to create with the drive to procreate, they believe that culture, generated by creativity, is another form of evolution. As people who procreate can alter our biological lineage, so those who create can alter the culture of civilizations. With that comes the necessity for social responsibility.

Creativity is a multifaceted phenomenon and humanity has a history of troubled times and great changes. Montuori, Combs, and Richards (2004) stress the importance of using creativity for the benefit of humanity, rather than its detriment. They state (p. 108), "Creativity is an extremely complex phenomenon. The paradoxical situation we find ourselves in is that creativity – the human capacity to bring something new into existence – is both our greatest hope and our greatest threat."

Evolution of Social and Creative Change: The Ratchet Effect and External Storage Devices

Civilization transforms not only through initial invention but also through continued innovation spurred by cultural interchange. This process of alterations over time, called the *ratchet-effect* (Tomasello et al., 1993, p. 495), is where each successive change uses the current object as a baseline to ratchet up an altered model. Ratcheted iterations over the centuries are what transformed a five-thousand-year-old Near Eastern hammered dulcimer into the modern grand piano (Peterson et al., 1994). Yet the ratchet effect is not limited to physical objects because creative ideas may also evolve through cultural interchange (Gabora & DiPaola, 2012). Ratcheted objects, which are the product of multiple stages, are also the result of a series of sequential creative trance states, where creativity is activated by something that inspires its own improvement.

A profound advance in human culture is the invention of external storage devices (Donald, 1995; Henshilwood et al., 2009). External memory aides, which include writing, ceremonial objects, counting systems, musical instruments, visual arts, graphic symbols, and other depictions and containers of information, vastly expand the capacity of the human internal or biological memory. Now virtual brain capacity is potentially the size of the internet with a virtual memory theoretically equal to storage in the digital cloud. In response, creative possibilities are expanding exponentially and with them, the parameters of our altered states. With new possibilities becoming increasingly available, who at this point, could predict or even imagine all the aspects of a postmodern creative trance?

CHAPTER 6

The Creative Trance and the Brain

The empires of the future are the empires of the mind
Winston Churchill

The great events of the world take place in the brain
Oscar Wilde

The mind is the seat of trance. The many ways that we think, consciously and unconsciously, shape our creative process and structure its creative trance. Every thought we have, every movement we make, changes the landscape of our brain by producing its own neural signature. By studying these accounts of the brain in action, contemporary neuroscience uncovers the neurological basis of creativity.

It also reveals the heterogeneity of creative trance states through their activation of different regions in the brain. Neural signatures of the creative trance can range from insights that solve everyday problems to the ecstatic states of Buddhist jhanas. While cognitive neuroscience is an extensive discipline with multiple connections to the creative process, this chapter will discuss selected aspects of neuroscience and their relationship to the creative trance.

Neuroscience: The Creative Trance and The Brain

Creative thinking is now being mapped electronically with fMRI scans (functional magnetic resonance imaging) and hdEED (high density electroencephalography) (Kounios & Beeman, 2015), as contemporary neuroscience brings us into a more neurologically transparent world. Neural signatures generating patterns of information are revealing the brain in action, creating visual traces of our thinking. Although neuroscience research does not use the term *creative trance*, it addresses multiple aspects of the creative process, such as generating and appreciating creative works, which this book identifies as a creative trance and an audience creative trance.

Throughout this chapter, we will see that creativity involves the capacity for contradictory ways of thinking that combine and synthesize into novel and useful results. Ellamil and associates (2012) found that creative people have a greater capacity for contradictory styles of thought and that creative thinking involves a unique assembly of neural processes not usually associated in ordinary cognition. While these processes may appear to be antithetical, in a creative trance they can combine into a paradoxical union of opposites (Jung, 1977), a whole greater than the sum of its parts.

Neuroscience and the Benefits of Creativity

The creative trance and the audience creative trance can bring a variety of health benefits. Singing and listening to music release endorphins, dopamine, serotonin, and oxytocin, brain neurotransmitters that are associated with happiness, bonding, and trust (Decker, 2019). Rhythmic music also promotes the release of endorphins (Tarr et al., 2014), which along with the body's endogenous opioid system facilitates social bonding and is associated with dancing, singing, listening to music, musical activities, synchronized sports, and laughter. When Clift and Morrison (2011) studied a group of small choirs in the United Kingdom, they found that regular group singing brought significant clinical improvement to people with serious chronic mental illness.

Loneliness and social isolation, which can bring mental and physical problems, are very prevalent in older adults. Yet they appear to be ameliorated through the experience of an audience creative trance. Using data from the *English Longitudinal Study of Ageing* (ELSA), Tymoszuk and associates (2019) found that while older adults benefitted from attending concerts, theatre, and the opera, they received a still greater protection against loneliness by going to galleries, exhibitions, and museums.

Creative arts are currently gaining wider acceptance as therapy to counteract loneliness (Decker, 2020). Montreal medical associations can now offer prescriptions for free admission to the Montreal Museum of Fine Arts in Quebec, and in the United Kingdom, there is a 2023 mental health initiative scheduled to allow physicians to prescribe visual art, dance, and singing lessons. In the United States, the Foundation for Art and Healing (2020) has its UnLonely Project, which sponsors the annual UnLonely Film Festival.

Creativity and the Default Mode Network

Creativity pervades our lives, and whenever our creative trance arises through daydreams and mind wanderings, we are accessing the default mode network (DMN) of our brain. Regarded as task-negative because it functions during times of rest, the DMN is comprised of five brain regions: the medial temporal lobes, the ventral and dorsal medial prefrontal cortex, the anterior lateral temporal cortex, the medial parietal regions, and the inferior parietal cortex with the temporoparietal junction (Abraham, 2018).

While creative thought takes place through multiple complex inter-actions among the major brain regions (Feist, 2010; Corballis, 2018), it can have a profound affiliation with the divergent thinking of the default mode network and the executive network (Mayseless et al., 2015; Marron & Faust, 2018). Yet there are variations. Limb and Braun (2008) found that when professional jazz pianists were improvising, their executive network indicated deactivation while their DMN showed activation.

The DMN is an inner-directed brain region and the place of our reveries, which are states of trance. This large brain network energizes when we disengage from our surroundings and turn inward (Kounios & Beeman, 2015). It becomes active during wakeful rest, those times during daydreaming, when our eyes are closed yet we are not asleep. Then our mind wanders, and our thoughts turn to ourselves, to past events, and future goals (Raichle et al., 2001; Raichle & Snyder, 2007). These inner experiences are the trance states of daily life, and they are frequent occurrences.

Our minds wander almost fifty percent of our waking hours (Corballis, 2018), and although mind wandering tends to occur when we are less happy (Killingsworth & Gilbert, 2010), it gives us greater access to creative ideas (Corballis, 2018). We can infer DMN activity in individuals like the physician and pharmacologist James Black (1924–2010). His predilection for reverie was a basis for the creativity that led to his 1988 Nobel Prize in Physiology or Medicine. "I daydream like mad," said Black (cited in Root-Bernstein & Root-Bernstein, 1999, p. 53), and described his thinking as "an imaginative sense, entirely open-ended and entirely pictorial."

The DMN, Openness to Experience, Exploration, and Dopamine

The DMN is associated with the personality trait of openness to experience (Richards, 2018), which encompasses the capacity to generate creative and imaginative ideas and the ability to engage in abstract thought. Beaty and associates (2016) believe there is a possible biological basis for openness to experience because they find the trait appears to facilitate efficient information processing in the DMN. An increased connection between the DMN and the inferior prefrontal cortex also indicates an ability to produce creative ideas (Beaty et al., 2014).

Kaufman and Gregoire (2016) link openness to experience with a drive for exploration and say the urge to explore may be the most important factor in creative achievement. Exploration, with its desire for novel information, has a neurological basis because the brain responds differently to the unfamiliar and the new. Every act of exploration arises from an individual's specific personality and unique neurophysiology. Kaufman and Gregoire call the neurotransmitter dopamine a neuromodulator of exploration because it promotes motivation and learning. By facilitating psychological plasticity, dopamine enhances flexible thinking and the cognitive strength to work with new behaviors and ideas. Through increasing our ability to engage with the unknown, it becomes a key to creativity and personal evolution.

Creativity and the Salience Network, Divergent and Convergent Thinking

Generative reverie in the DMN is only part of the creative process because insights must be communicated. James Black had to translate his imaginative imagery into the mathematics, diagrams, and words of analytical pharmacology. To do this, one must transition from the divergent, open, creative thought of the DMN to the convergent, closed, evaluative thought that activates the fronto-singulo-parietal Central Executive Network (CEN). The CEN is a large group of brain regions that focus on cognitive control and goal-directed activity (Abraham, 2018). The brain region that mediates the transitions between the DMN and the CEN is the salience network, which includes the orbital frontoinsular cortices and the dorsal anterior cingulate (Goulden et al., 2014; Abraham, 2018).

Both divergent and convergent thinking are necessary for successful creativity and both are operative in the creative trance. The divergent imaginative, open, visionary, intuitive, spontaneous generation of ideas melds with the convergent logical, goal-directed, deliberate, concrete, analytical thinking to generate original concepts with workable solutions. Creativity's neurological melding of divergent and convergent thinking is like the fusion of opposites in a personality uniting to create a higher level of functioning. While Jung (1977) wrote about this dynamic as a path to personality integration, the activation of convergent and divergent thinking in creativity leads to the integrative work of generating an original yet workable product.

Brain Sites for Generation and Evaluation of Everyday Creativity

Creativity is an amalgam of generation and evaluation that takes place at multiple sites in the brain. As Mayseless and associates (2015, p. 232) say, "Original ideas are a product of the interaction between a system that generates ideas and a control system that evaluates these ideas." They add that to achieve creative outcomes, it is not only necessary to generate new ideas but also to guard against predictable solutions.

In their study on divergent thinking in everyday creativity, Mayseless and associates found that generating original ideas and novel connections, while avoiding conventional thinking, activates the medial prefrontal cortex (mPFC) and the posterior cingulate cortex of the DMN, while evaluation activates the ventral anterior cingulate cortex. Although their study focused on everyday creativity, they suggest that eminent creativity may be generated by people whose brains show extremely high connectivity between the inferior parietal regions and the anterior cingulate cortex.

Brain Sites for Generation and Evaluation of Visual Art

In their research on the generation and evaluation of visual art, Ellamil and associates (2012) also identified multiple sites for creativity in the brain. They had art students design book cover illustrations inside an fMRI scanner, using an fMRI-compatible tablet. The students followed a set protocol that directed them to separate and alternate between the generative and evaluative aspects of their creative process. In their creative generation, the students appeared to access images and inspiration from their memories, activating the medial temporal lobe memory network with its hippocampus and parahippocampus.

The default mode network appeared to be active during generative creativity because of its low cognitive control. Yet it was also active, along with the salience network, in evaluative creativity through its role in visceral and affective responses. The executive network, with its high cognitive control and capacity for focusing on details, appeared to activate in response to the analytical assessments necessary during evaluative creativity.

Brain Sites for Generation and Evaluation of Poetry

When Liu and associates (2015) examined the generation of poetry with its evaluations and revisions, they also wanted to investigate the influence of expertise. Liu and associates found that in both novices and experts the medial prefrontal cortex (MPFC) was active in generating poems and in evaluating/revising them. Although their small sample size did not include eminent poets, they found marked differences in cognitive control between novices and more experienced writers.

While generating poetry, the experts exhibited significantly less activation of the dorsolateral prefrontal system and the parietal executive system, indicating a greater suspension of cognitive control than the novices. This suggests that in their creative trance, the experts were able to maintain a more open mind during generation, casting wider mental nets for outlying sparks of originality. The cognitive control that was lessened during generation was then reinstated during revision. Liu and associates hypothesize (p. 3369) that "extremely skilled, true genius might be characterized by a unique and discontinuous neural architecture" and suggest that this be the subject of future studies.

Creativity and the Brain Hemispheres

The right and left hemispheres of the brain are both active in the creative process. Their difference in function was known in the nineteenth century with the work of Broca, who discovered a location for speech in the left hemisphere of the brain, now known as Broca's area, and the research of Charcot and Janet, who attributed hysteria to problems in the right hemisphere (Corballis, 2018).

Public interest in brain hemisphere function was ignited in the mid-twentieth century with the work of Sperry and Gazzaniga, who operated on patients with severe epilepsy to stop their previously intractable seizures (Gazzaniga et al., 1962; Sperry, 1982). By surgically severing the brain's corpus callosum, which is a thick band of nerve tissue that both separates and connects the right and left hemispheres, Sperry and Gazzaniga not only reduced the epileptic seizures but also realized they could now study the hemispheres independently.

Their initial discoveries that the left hemisphere was the center of speech and the right hemisphere was the source of visual and nonverbal abilities entered public awareness and resulted in a widespread idealization of the right hemisphere as the sole center of creativity. While subsequent research finds an interplay between the two hemispheres with both sides of the brain contributing to the creative process (Whitman et al., 2010; Lindell, 2011; Corballis, 2018), visual art maintains a strong connection to the right hemisphere (Miller & Hou, 2004).

Flashes of Insight in the Creative Trance

Flashes of insight are some of the most dramatic moments in a creative trance, facilitating immediate shifts in our knowledge, work, and emotions. They range from the problem-solving insights of daily life to the profound flashes of illumination in a creative or religious experience. Friedrich Nietzsche (2017/1888, p. 47) described the experience of insight as "a thought suddenly flashes up like lightning, it comes with necessity, without faltering – I never had any choice in the matter." Likewise, the poet Remy de Gourmont (1858–1915) stated, "My conceptions rise into the field of consciousness like a flash of lightning or the flight of a bird" (cited in Wallas, 1926, p. 80). Yet these insights, which seem to arise full blown into awareness, may be the workings of the unconscious mind erupting into conscious thought.

Before the moment of insight, a briefly idling section in the back of the brain shifts into alpha, flaring into what the neuroscientists Kounios and Beeman (2015, pp. 84–85) call the "Alpha Brain Blink." This paves the way for the right temporal lobe, which fires into gamma rhythms producing a "Gamma Insight Burst" with a conscious solution to the problem. Kounios and Beeman (2015, p. 212) note that "just before viewing a problem that participants would eventually solve with insight, they disengaged from their surroundings and directed their attention inwardly on their own thoughts."

The poet William Wordsworth (1770–1850) wrote about this creative eruption from quiet (1985/1895, p. 82), saying that "poetry is the spontaneous overflow of powerful feelings; it takes its origin from emotion recollected in tranquility." Wordsworth believed his poetry had a foundation in memory, and Dietrich (2004) suggests that creative insights are mediated by neural circuits terminating at the working memory buffer in the prefrontal cortex.

"Insightfuls" and "Analysts" in the Creative Trance

When Kounios and Beeman (2015) recorded the electroencephalograms (EEG) of people in a resting state and then while they were solving problems, they found two distinct patterns of problem-solving. One group tended to have more insights and use their insights to solve problems, while the other group generated solutions to a problem in an organized and systematic step-by-step procedure. Although Kounios and Beeman note that most individuals use both methods to differing degrees, they called the more insightful group the Insightfuls and the more analytic group the Analysts. Highly creative Insightfuls have diffuse unfocused attention that allows a greater input of environmental stimuli, while the more logical Analysts have a narrower, more directed focus of attention permitting less environmental stimuli.

For those, who want to increase their insightful aspect, Subramaniam and associates (2009) find positive moods help generate insights and solve creative problems. Yet not everyone solves problems with dramatic insight. Some people succeed through persistence, and their continued deliberation can produce its own type of creative trance. In his essay *The Making of a Poem* (1985/1946), the poet Stephen Spender (1909–1995) said he worked this way and lamented the enormous amount of effort it took to write his poems. Referring to one of his notebooks that was begun in 1944, he says (1985/1946, p. 116), "About a hundred pages of it are covered with writing, and from this have emerged about six poems."

Patterns of Thought and Resting-State Brain Waves

There is a relationship between personality, creativity, and brain structure (Vartanian, 2018). Insightfuls and Analysts not only think differently but they have different resting-state brain activity, and their resting-states correspond to their method of problem-solving (Kounios et al., 2008; Kounios & Beeman, 2015). Resting-state brain waves, which, are highly influenced by brain structure and genetics, appear to be relatively constant over time. Spectral analyses of resting-states showed that highly creative people have more right brain hemisphere activation, with activity at the right dorsal frontal, the right inferior frontal, and the right parietal regions.

In contrast, analytical people have more activation in the left hemisphere with activity at the left inferior frontal and the left anterior temporal regions. Another difference is that Insightfuls have more activity in their visual cortex than Analysts (Kounios et al., 2008). Data revealed that Insightfuls have lower occipital alpha-band activity resulting in less inhibition of the resting-state visual system, suggesting active visual information processing, and possibly the visualization aspect of a creative trance.

Analysts have a higher occipital beta activity, indicating there is a heightened focus of attention.

Combining Insight and Analysis in the Creative Trance

Just as convergent and divergent thought are both necessary for creativity, so are the capacities for insight and analysis. While Kounios and Beeman note that most individuals can and do use the two methods in varying degrees, the poet Stephen Spender (1909–1995) finds both are integral to the creative process. He identifies them (1985/1946, p. 115) as "two types of concentration: one is immediate and complete, the other is plodding and only completed by stages."

Acknowledging that "genius works in different ways to achieve its ends" (p. 116), Spender contrasts the examples of Mozart, who composed music entirely in his head and then transcribed the completed compositions onto paper, with Beethoven, who began with fragments of themes copied into notebooks that he would work on for years. Spender notes that some of Beethoven's initial ideas were so clumsy that musicologists were amazed at how they developed into extraordinary music. Referring to his own struggles with writing, Spender says that (p. 119) "everything in poetry is work except inspiration" and cites the poet Paul Valéry's (1871–1945) concept of inspiration as "One line is given to the poet by God or nature, the rest he has to discover by himself."

Top-Down versus Bottom-Up Information Processing and Attentional States

Another cognitive dichotomy in creativity is top-down versus bottom-up information processing (Kounios & Beeman, 2015; Abraham, 2018). Yet like the other dualisms, it is their dynamic combination that describes and augments creative output. In the creative process, bottom-up information processing is sensory driven, activated by stimuli in the environment at that moment, while top-down processing is concept-driven and controlled by the frontal lobe. Top-down information organizes our thoughts and emotions, focusing on what is important, and categorizing stimuli for more rapid brain processing.

Yet creativity depends on novelty and can wither in overcontrol and extended categorization. That is why Abraham (2018) notes that insufficiencies in top-down control can be fortuitous to creativity. With fewer restrictions, the mind has greater access to raw sensory information and the possibilities of new combinations, cognitive disinhibition, and unusual perspectives that enhance the creative process. This leads to the unexpected and the surprises in a creative work that make it more memorable.

Vartanian (2009) finds there are a variety of attentional states in the creative process, employed as strategies in response to task demands, indicating attention is variable and adjustable rather than a steady trait. In the early stages of problem-solving when a task may be ambiguous or ill-defined, there may be defocused attention that results in slower brain processing. Yet a strategy for the later stages of problem-solving, with well-defined tasks, may be focused attention with its faster processing of less ambiguous situations. Both types of attention can manifest in a creative trance.

The Interrupted Creative Trance

Like a butterfly migrating thousands of miles on tissue-thin wings, the mental range of a creative trance can be far reaching yet fragile. Sometimes when interrupted, a trance state may never be regained. Perhaps the most famous interruption was when the poet Samuel Taylor Coleridge (1772–1834) had a business visitor from Porlock. Coleridge (1985) had seen a vision of the complete poem of *Kublai Khan* in his mind and had just begun to transcribe it. Yet over an hour later when the man left, the trance state with its poetry had also vanished. Possibly Coleridge, who had his initial vision on a medication that he was given, was not able to retrieve the vision an hour later when the effects of the medication may have lessened, indicating that the inspiration might have been encoded as a state-specific memory.

More common interruptions to the creative trance are usually noise and environmental distractions. There appears to be a widespread tendency among creative people to have a hypersensitivity to sound (Kasof, 1997; Zabelina et al., 2015, Kaufman & Gregoire, 2016). The writer Marcel Proust (1871–1922), who had difficulty screening out environmental noise, kept the blinds drawn in his bedroom where he worked, lined the walls with cork, and wore earplugs while writing. The scientist Charles Darwin (1809–1882) said that sounds other people did not even notice bothered him. In response, he moved to a very secluded home that was extremely quiet. The composer Edward Elgar (1857–1934) also moved away to find silence. He found an isolated country cottage that provided the necessary quiet and solitude.

In his essay *On Noise* (2013/1851), the philosopher Arthur Schopenhauer (1788–1860) revealed that he was chronically unable to filter out environmental sounds. For Schopenhauer, a man with great compassion for nonhuman animals (2014/1840), the most painful and intrusive sounds he heard from the street outside his home was the cracking of whips on horses. Lamenting that noise upset him and interrupted his concentration, Schopenhauer found other eminent creative people, such as the philosopher Immanuel Kant (1234–1804) and the writer Johann Goethe (1749–1832), who also had difficulty with unwanted sound.

"Leaky" Sensory Gating and the Creative Trance

Current neuroscience is proving Schopenhauer to be correct. Zabelina and associates (2015, p. 77) find that creative people have "'leaky' sensory gating," which makes it difficult for them to screen out environmental sounds, while less creative people with stronger sensory filters are not as impacted by noise. They measured sensory gating by EEG data, electrophysiological recordings, using the P50 ERP, an event-related potential that indicates the degree of response to a stimulus given fifty milliseconds after an initial stimulus (Yadon, et al., 2009). Here the stimuli were two auditory clicks heard with a headset, and the degree that the second click was inhibited or habituated relative to the first was the neural marker for sensory gating.

   Zabelina and associates not only found creative people were less able to screen out the second auditory click, indicating they had leaky sensory filters, but also discovered that the more creative accomplishments a person had, the leakier the sensory gating. Leaky sensory filters indicate lower latent inhibition with a reduced ability to ignore extraneous stimuli. Yet this seeming incapacity is integral to the creative process and its trance. By allowing many stimuli to enter, leaky sensors generate a greater breadth of possibilities leading to increased information processing. While leaky sensors may sometimes cause distractions, they may also bring previously peripheral ideas into central focus for unexpected creative solutions.

Synesthesia and the Creative Trance

People who have synesthesia may be able to hear colors while seeing them and see sounds while hearing them, and it structures their creative trance. Known as synesthetes, they may also taste sounds, feel sounds on the skin, hear odors, hear images, taste images, and see numbers, letters, months, years, and days in color. There is also mirror-touch synesthesia, where people perceive touch to another person's body as if it were their own (Banissy, 2013). In all, there are more than one hundred types of synesthesia (Ramachandran & Hubbard, 2005).

These connections can occur because synesthesia is an automatic cross-modal neurological response (Cytowic, 2002, 2018; van Campen, 2008; Banissy, 2013; Simmonds-Moore, 2020). It happens when a stimulus to one sensory pathway in the brain (the inducer) simultaneously activates an additional sensory pathway (the concurrent) to produce a conscious experience of two attributes not usually joined together. While synesthesia may arise after an injury, it is usually a genetic condition that appears in families (Simner & Carmichael, 2015).

Synesthetes as Creative Individuals

The novelist Vladimir Nabokov (1899–1977) was a synesthete as were his mother and son (van Campen, 2008). The experience of synesthesia may increase in a creative trance, because imagining an object can produce a greater synesthetic response than physically seeing it (Ramachandran & Hubbard, 2005). There are quantified associations between creativity and synesthesia with synesthetes testing higher on the traits of openness and absorption, showing increased use of mental imagery, and having better verbal comprehension (Chun & Hupe 2016).

Synesthetes are also more likely to be in creative occupations and use synesthetic experiences as integral to their creative trance. The actor Marilyn Monroe (1926–1962) was a synesthete (Mailer, 1973), as were her sister and niece, who said Monroe used her synesthesia as an ability she combined with acting techniques (Seaberg, 2012). The visual artist Vasily Kandinsky (1866–1944) experienced colors as their attributes, such as sticky, rough, smooth, sharp, hard, soft, or dry (Kandinsky, 1977). He used these synesthetic responses as a basis for his color theory and his paintings.

Van Campen (2008) cites three composers, Olivier Messiaen, György Ligeti, and Michael Torke, whose synesthesia is central to their creative trance. Olivier Messiaen (1908–1992) saw and heard music in colors and organized his works with musical modes corresponding to their color images. For György Ligeti (1923–2006), sound, image, and touch were interposed, and since childhood he imagined music as pictures. Michael Torke (b. 1961), who sees sounds in color, as well as letters, months, days, and years, uses his synesthesia as a source of inspiration for composing.

Grapheme-Color Synesthetes and Their Creative Trance

The most common kind of synesthesia is grapheme-color synesthesia, which is the experience of seeing letters and numbers in colors (Cytowic, 2002, 2018; van Campen, 2008). A letter *A* might be red and a number *7* may be green, and while different synesthetes will see different colors, the associations of the specific color with a specific grapheme will remain constant throughout a lifetime. The writer Vladimir Nabokov, the physicist Richard Feynman (1918–1988), and the chemist Monona Rossol (b. 1936) are all grapheme-color synesthetes.

Nabokov had characters in his novels with synesthesia and said the letter *A* appeared in different colors ranging from black to gray in the four languages that he spoke (van Campen, 2008). Feynman (2001) saw the letters and mathematical functions of his equations in colors, and Rossol taught herself to read using synesthesia (Zausner, 2016). Severely dyslexic as a child, Rossol realized that if she saw letters and numbers as their colors, they stopped moving around and became anchored on the page, allowing her to read and do mathematics.

Synesthetic Brains: Greater Connectivity and the Capacity for Metaphor

FMRI scans of grapheme-color synesthetes suggest they have a greater connectivity between the auditory areas of the brain and the visual regions, specifically the color region, V4 (Dovern et al., 2012). The strength of a synesthetic response appears to correlate with the degree of connectivity between the right frontoparietal, visual, and auditory regions in the brain. Diffusion Tensor Imaging of synesthetes' brains indicates structural hyperconnectivity in multiple brain areas, suggesting a difference in functioning from non-synesthete brains (Rouw, 2013). The hyperconnectivity in the brains of synesthetes may be related to their increased creativity (Mulvenna, 2007, 2013) and possibly to a stronger memory (Heyrman, 2005; Meir & Rothen, 2013).

Ramachandran and Hubbard (2005) believe that the human capacity for synesthesia may be neurologically connected with the capacity for metaphor, a widespread aptitude in creative people. They also suggest that this linkage may have facilitated the ability for abstract thought. Noting that both metaphor and synesthesia join seemingly unrelated items, a propensity central to creativity, they postulate that this cross-modal synthesis arises in multiple parts of the brain. These regions include the junction of the temporal, parietal, and occipital lobes and in the angular gyrus contained within it, as well as in the fusiform gyrus, and the V4 color area. They believe that cross-modal connections may have opened the way for more complex levels of abstract thought. We may all be synesthetes to some degree (Van Campen, 2010).

Spontaneous Synesthesia versus Intentional/Metaphoric Synesthesia

In addition to the spontaneous synesthesia that arises unintentionally from cross-modal neural connections, there are intentionally generated synesthetic experiences. They are used metaphorically with abstract thinking and appear to be the product of a creative trance. The first type may be considered *spontaneous synesthesia* and the second type *intentional/metaphorical synesthesia*.

When the visual artist Anne Theresa Adams (1940–2007) interpreted the music of Ravel's *Bolero* as a painting, *Unravelling Bolero,* by consciously choosing colors to match its sounds, she did not report classic synesthesia (Seeley et al., 2008). Instead of involuntarily seeing colors while hearing the notes, Adams created the sound/color associations intentionally before rendering them in paint. This voluntary metaphoric interpretation appears to be a deliberate self-induced empathic type of synesthesia. It occurs when creative people intentionally create a synesthetic response during the creative trance. They may sense this as an embodied visceral experience by *feeling* their choice through empathically projecting a part of themselves into the work.

Intentional/Metaphoric Synesthesia across Domains

Intentional metaphoric synesthesia manifests across domains, and as Van Campen (2013, pp. 631–646) notes, "artists use less strict definitions of synesthesia than scientists." Intentional metaphoric synesthesia is evident in Piet Mondrian's (1872–1944) painting *Broadway Boogie Woogie* (1942–1943), a visual interpretation of jazz as brightly colored squares spaced on a grid suggesting the streets of Manhattan. Metaphorical synesthesia occurs when composers deliberately identify personages with a composite of notes, such as Richard Wagner's (1813–1883) *Ride of the Valkyrie* from his 1856 opera *Die Walküre* and Igor Stravinsky's (1882–1971) entrance of the *Firebird* in his 1910 ballet *The Firebird.*

There may also be a type of metaphorical synesthesia present in the embodiment aspect of a performance. Here, instead of experiencing music as colors, the body is intentionally experienced as a different being. It occurs in the ballerina becoming a swan in the ballet *Swan Lake* and in the actor playing a historic person in a Kabuki drama. It is also in the martial artist assuming a fused identity with the animal from which her moves are derived, such as the crane in *Soaring Crane Qiqong*.

While this experience can be viewed as an empathic projection of the self into an art form during a creative trance, it may also be considered as a type of metaphorical mirror-touch synesthesia because of its similarities to actual mirror-touch synesthesia. In both states body-to-body physical correspondences are empathically connected with a blurred line between self and other. While in actual mirror-touch synesthesia the other is a different person, in metaphorical mirror-touch synesthesia the other is an intentionally transformed self.

Neuroscience of Meditation: Transcendent States and Beneficial Neuroplasticity

Meditation is an ancient practice that has become increasingly popular in our hectic modern world. Beginning with calm and focus, meditative practices may escalate to a place beyond trance, reaching a sense of the ineffable. By studying the brain during transcendent meditative states, neuroscience is providing a venerable tradition with a new technological dimension. The creative trance of meditation does not focus on generating a poem or a sonata, but on recreating and transforming the self. I have been meditating since 1973, and it has changed my life for the better. Current neuroscience is validating this self-evolution through examples of meditation-induced neuroplasticity.

Long-term Tibetan Buddhist meditators appear to change the functioning of their brain in multiple ways (Lutz et al., 2004; Davidson & Lutz, 2008). They have less activation in the amygdala, suggesting a decreased response to emotionally charged stimuli and a greater ability to concentrate. During their meditative practice of boundless compassion, the Tibetan monks produced high-amplitude gamma waves that appear to promote neural synchrony and more effective brain functioning. This transcendent level of compassion, known as *"uncontrived spontaneous great compassion"* (Houshmand et al., 2002p. 15), is a direct response to suffering without involving sadness as a transitional stage.

Research on other long-term meditators found that meditation can thicken the prefrontal cortex and the right anterior insula, brain areas for sensory processing, attention, and body awareness, and may also reduce cortical thinning due to age (Lazar et al., 2005). Long-term meditators also show significantly increased gray matter in their right orbito-frontal cortex and right hippocampus, both regions associated with emotional regulation (Luders et al., 2009). They can also evidence greater structural connectivity throughout the brain (Luders et al., 2011).

Multiple Modes of Meditation and Their Neural Signatures

In 2008 Lutz and associates divided some standard meditative practices into two categories: *focused attention*, where attention is sustained on an object, usually the breath, and *open monitoring*, a nonreactive awareness without explicit focus, as seen in mindfulness meditations. Travis and Shear (2010, p. 1110) propose a third category they call *automatic self-transcending* meditation, which uses "techniques designed to transcend their own activity." This would include repeating a mantra to ascend to higher states of consciousness.

Using an EEG, Travis and Shear (2010) found that all three categories have specific neural signatures. Focused attention, which is part of the Buddhist and Chinese meditative cultures, produced beta/gamma activity. Open monitoring, a meditative practice used in the Hindu/Vedic, Chinese, and Buddhist traditions, produced theta activity, while automatic self-transcending meditations of the Chinese and Hindu/Vedic cultures produced alpha activity. Alpha waves are also a neural signature of transcendental meditation, which derives from the Hindu/Vedic tradition (Travis & Wallace, 1999).

All these types of meditation can be initiated for health and as the practice deepens they may advance beyond trance to transcendent states. Yet there appears to be more than these three categories. There is the neuroscience study of Catholic Carmelite nuns, who reexperienced their mystical union with God (Beauregard & Paquette, 2006; Beauregard & O'Leary, 2007). Results from fMRI and quantitative electroencephalography indicated increased activation in multiple brain sites, including the visual cortex, indicating visualization, and the mesial temporal cortex, which the researchers suggest might be associated with the subjective feeling of communing with a spiritual reality. The nuns also had significantly higher theta activity during their mystical experience relative to their resting states.

Buddhist Meditation on the Four Jhanas

In Buddhism, meditation on the four Jhanas is known for its generation of joy. These four steps of ecstatic release from the material world unfold from within each other on the way to a non-dual consciousness of enlightenment (Brahmavamso, 2005). Using fMRI and hdEED, Hagerty and associates (2013) found that brain changes began quickly after an experienced meditator entered the Jhanas and saw variances in the states of the different Jhanas.

Activation in the meditator's cortical processes and nucleus accumbens of the dopamine/opioid reward region suggested extreme joy. Yet they occurred with below resting state readings in brain sites related to orientation, verbalization, and external awareness. That the meditator's reward system was activated without imagined movements or physical cues led Hagerty and associates (p. 11) to conclude that the "Jhana's reduced sense awareness is not incidental to achieving extreme pleasure but is a contributing condition."

Meditations That Open to Transcendence

Many meditations open to the path of transcendence. They include the Taoist circulation of energy through the meridians and the Yoga concentration on chakras (Travis & Shear, 2010). There is also the meditative journey of ascent through the heavens taken by Merkabah mystics in Judaism (Scholem, 1987) and an ecstatic union with the divine in the Sufi tradition of Islam (Markoff, 2016). The existence of multiple pathways to the ineffable has been known for centuries across cultures. It is intimated by the Zen Master Mumon, also known as Ekai (1183–1260), in his koan *The Gateless Gate* (2008, p. x):

> The Great Way has no gates
> Thousands of roads enter it
> When one passes through this gateless gate,
> One walks freely between heaven and earth

These pathways are not only cultural routes; they are also the individual attempts of sentient beings throughout time. As their ongoing numbers increase, they will continue toward boundlessness, like the transcendence that is their goal.

CHAPTER 7

Dynamics of the Creative Trance

In all chaos there is a cosmos, in all disorder, a secret order

Carl Jung

One must have chaos within oneself to give birth to a dancing star

Friedrich Nietzsche

Nonlinearity with its capacity for growth and change defines our lives, our thoughts, and the universe in which we live. By revealing the underlying patterns of cognition and behavior, nonlinear dynamics describes the creative trance as a creative chaos (Macdonald, 1990; Zausner, 1996, 2016), capable of originality, transformation, and bringing forth the new. With its disciplines of chaos theory and complexity theory, nonlinear dynamics provides models to understand our unpredictable, unrepeatable, yet ever-evolving existence in a constantly changing world. It studies processes that never exactly duplicate themselves or progress in a straight line, and although they may seem disorderly instead contain a dynamic order capable of growth and change (Prigogine & Stengers, 1984; Nicolis & Prigogine, 1989; Zausner, 1996; Schuldberg, 1999).

Creative People and the Nonlinear Chaos of Creativity

Intuitively resonating with the nonlinear far-from-equilibrium state of chaos, creative people may see it as intrinsic to their work. The novelist and essayist James Baldwin (1924–1987), who calls the creative person an "incorrigible disturber of the peace" (1962, p. 17), insisted that (p. 18) "The artist must know, and he must let us know, that there is nothing stable under heaven."

Describing her writing, Hilary Mantel (b. 1952) says it is always "off balance ... never in equilibrium" (cited in Currey, 2019, p. 227), and that writing "makes for a life that by its very nature, has to be unstable." Yet she warns that "if it ever became stable, you'd be finished." Selected from the large science of nonlinear dynamics, the examples in this chapter are not presented mathematically but as metaphorical models that correlate with and help us understand our psychological processes and the creative trance.

Nonlinear Dynamics: Chaos Theory, Complexity Theory, and the Creative Trance

As nonlinear beings living in a nonlinear world, it is understandable that our states of creative trance can be modeled by nonlinear dynamics (Zausner, 2022). Older worldviews, such as the Newtonian model, described a clockwork universe, mechanized, orderly, and predictable. Daily life constantly reminds us that this is not true. Instead, we live in an unpredictable world, but it is the multiple variables and constant surprises in our world and in ourselves that bring change. Newtonian dynamics concerns the linear interaction of only two variables, yet our lives are vastly more complex. In his mathematics, Henri Poincare (1854–1912) demonstrated that the interaction of three or more variables creates a nonlinear event (Moeckel, 2012). Known as the three-body or n-body problem, it is a basis for chaos theory, where multiple interactions can introduce the formation of new order.

Multiple interactions make the creative process a complex system, and the study of these nonlinear systems is called complexity theory (Galanter, 2003). Here, multiple variables organize themselves through structure and pattern into a dynamic whole far beyond the sum of its parts and capable of initiating an emergent order (Nicolis & Prigogine, 1989; Waldrop, 1992). We see this dynamic in a creative trance where many possibilities interact with each other, with the creative person, the culture, and the environment, creating the emerging order of an original work. Consciousness itself may be an emergent phenomenon and dreams may be an emergent phenomenon of our consciousness (Krippner & Combs, 2000).

Chaos: Generating Creativity and the New

With its multiple interacting variables, the creative chaos is not a disorder but a deterministic or generative chaos that leads to new order (Prigogine & Stengers, 1984; Zausner, 1996, 2022). The multiple possibilities arising in the chaos of a creative trance may conceivably be in a type of quantum superposition until they self-organize into a resolution (Gabora, 2017). The connection between chaos and the new is ancient and evident in the chaotic celebrations that bring in the New Year. It is also a part of religious traditions such as the Judeo-Christian Bible (Genesis 1:2), where the world begins in chaos, and in the Hindu Rig Veda (RV 10.121) where the *Hiranyagarbha*, the golden egg of creation, floats on the primeval waters of chaos.

Instinctively realizing the connection between chaos and generation, creative people may enhance their creative trance with an environmental chaos such as a thunderstorm. Acknowledging that everything begins in chaos in the Preface to her novel *Frankenstein* (1994), Mary Shelley (1797–1851) wrote the book during a thunderstorm and brought her creature to life with a lightning bolt. Charles Burchfield (1893–1967) found that painting during the chaos of a thunderstorm heightened his creative process. Having just set up his easel when a storm came, Burchfield refused to stop painting. Instead, he worked "with thunder crashing, boughs breaking, and rain falling in torrents. A glorious few hours when I seemed to become one of the elements" (cited in Eliot, 1957, p. 236).

Unpredictability, Struggles, Risks, and Breakthrough Bifurcations

The nonlinearity of the creative process is driven by the chaos of the unconscious mind. This wrests the work away from illusions of rational conscious control or predictability. Even when a creative trance may not seem externally chaotic, it is a state of high energy. Creative people appear to acknowledge and respect the nonlinearity inherent in their work and accept its unpredictable nature.

As Stewart (2002, p. 318) noted about the visual artist Willem de Kooning (1904–1997), "Always an intuitive painter, de Kooning often said that if he knew where he was going in a painting, he was going in the wrong direction." The writer E. L. Doctorow (1931–2015) also recognized the impossibility of knowing the long-term outcome of his creative works. He explained that (1988, p. 305) "Writing a novel is like driving a car at night. You can only see as far as your headlights, but you can make the whole trip that way."

As nonlinear occurrences, creative works can never be exactly duplicated, and their chaotic elements may be accentuated through risk taking. Yet this keeps the work vibrant. The pianist Vladimir Horowitz (1903–1989) said he never played a piece of music in the same way twice, acknowledging "because it is always different, it is always new" (cited in Mach, 1991, p. 119). Horowitz also believed in risk taking and said (p. 117) that a creative person should "never be afraid to take risks."

Another nonlinear aspect of creativity is the chaotic struggle that leads to a breakthrough. In nonlinear dynamics, breakthroughs can be modeled as bifurcations, occurring when the energy in a system increases until it bifurcates to the next level. In the creative process, this energy may arise while working on a problem until its solution breaks through into conscious awareness as a flash of insight. The contralto Marian Anderson (1897–1993), who described music as "an elusive thing" (cited in Currey, 2019, pp. 88–89), stated she would struggle intensely on a song without appearing to make progress. Then "suddenly," said Anderson, "there is a flash of understanding. What has appeared useless labor for days becomes fruitful at an unpredictable moment."

Attractors and Fractals

Not only are we nonlinear systems but the mind, our consciousness, is also nonlinear (Krippner & Combs, 2000) and has multiple interacting components that progress in time (Abraham, 2016). A characteristic of nonlinear systems is that they evolve toward attractors, which can be an active boundary containing the system or a basin of attraction which functions as a goal (Abraham et al., 1989). Psychologically, our belief systems act as attractors (Goertzel, 1995), shaping our lives and even organizing our perceptions.

Nonlinear systems also have a fractal nature. Fractals are self-similar patterns that repeat in space and time with a scale invariant complexity, which means they look similar despite a difference in size (Mandelbrot, 1983). Fractals are found in the repeating pattens of natural structures such as waves in the ocean, daisies in a field, and peas in a pod. Mathematically created geometric fractals like the Koch snowflake, which is comprised of repeating triangles, can be regular and exact, but in the natural world they vary. The leaves of a tree are similar but not identical, yet they are in a fractal relationship with each other.

In art, fractal structures can be either exact or approximate (Zausner, 1996, 2022; Taylor, 2004). Fractals can occur in repeated elements within a work, when works are in a series, and in the fractal relationship of the finished product to the intention of the creator. There also appears to be an interconnected fractal basis for our consciousness (Pincus et al., 2019). Yet here, fractal thought patterns and their psychologically motivated actions contain a similarity of meaning rather than imagery. Repeated thoughts and actions have a fractal quality as do transference and countertransference when we overlay a past personal experience onto someone in the present.

Attractors, Fractals, and Two Physicists

Although usually unconscious, transference was a conscious awareness in the creative process of the physicist Richard Feynman (1918–1988). When living in California, Feynman went to a weekly sketch class that the psychologist Terry Marks-Tarlow also attended. She wrote (2008, p. 166), "He confessed to me in private that his love for his first wife Arline was so great that he continually sought shadows of her features in the face of every woman he drew." Arline, who died at age twenty-five from lymphatic tuberculosis, was the love of Feynman's life and his grief for her was unending. Generated through the ongoing energies of love and longing, Arline was the attractor in Feynman's nonlinear creative trance, and her face became a repeating fractal image in his art. Memory has a fractal aspect because it creates a cognitive construct that matches the remembered actuality.

Love and grief also propelled the creative trance of physicist Ronald Lawrence Mallett (b. 1945). The attractor was his great longing to see his father again. His father died of a heart attack when Mallett was age ten. This intense desire turned Mallett (2006) toward the scientific possibility of time travel, an idea that was inspired by two creative trances in childhood. The first trance came at age twelve when he was transfixed by an illustration for *The Time Machine* by H. G. Wells. Mallet tried to build an apparatus like the one in the story, using old television tubes and pipes, but his machine stayed in the present. The second creative trance came shortly afterward when Mallet became enthralled by Einstein's concept of time as a fourth dimension and the effects of motion on time. Carrying his fascination with time travel and relativity theory into adulthood, Mallett (2000, 2003) became a theoretical physicist, researching the effects of circulating laser light on the properties of space-time.

Dissipative Structures and Strange Attractors

In nonlinear dynamics, human beings can be modeled as nonequilibrium dissipative structures (Zausner, 1996, p. 202). These are adaptive nonlinear systems that constantly respond to environmental or inner stimuli by taking in and discharging energy, while maintaining the integrity of themselves (Prigogine & Stengers, 1984). Nonliving systems, like the

Great Red Spot, an anticyclonic storm on the planet Jupiter, can also be dissipative structures (Briggs & Peat, 1989). This mass of swirling winds larger than our planet Earth is constantly taking in and releasing energy, while existing for hundreds of years within the boundaries of its strange attractor. Chaotic systems are contained within strange attractors, dynamic parameters that are never exact and never exactly repeatable, like the boundaries of our nonlinear mind (Zausner, 2020). We continually take in new information and discharge unnecessary concepts in an ongoing interchange with our environment that fuels self-evolution while maintaining the self.

These adaptive interchanges occur when perseverance in the creative trance turns adequacy into excellence. Using eminent role models as attractors, athletes and dancers perfect their form by training intensely. During their quest for achievement, they assimilate new methods and judge the accuracy of criticisms. By keeping what is beneficial and discarding the rest, they maintain the essence of themselves.

Self-Organization and Emergence

Complex nonlinear systems have the capacity for self-transformation through self-organization, a seemingly spontaneous process where local parts of a system interact to generate greater complexity and the emergence of a new global order (Prigogine & Stengers, 1984). This dynamic can occur in the creative trance, a state that facilitates emergence. It happens metaphorically when notes combine into a symphony, when words and ideas produce a narrative, when dance steps meld into a choreography, and when brushstrokes build a painting (Zausner, 2022). The visual artist Georgie O'Keeffe (1887–1986) regards her work as self-organizing. "The color grew as I painted," she said. "My paintings sometimes grow by pieces from what is around" (1976).

Human beings are complex self-organizing systems (Pincus et al., 2019), capable of transforming and recreating themselves. Self-evolution is inherent in human nature with its teleological drive to evolve from infancy to maturity. The process of psychological maturity may accelerate through meditation when quieting the mind from internal dialogue promotes states of spontaneous self-organization (Hunt, 1995). We have new order constantly emerging in response to ongoing daily events along with multiple opportunities to set a new course. Every thought changes the landscape of our mind and our reactions can alter the trajectory of a life.

The Butterfly Effect: Sensitivity to Initial Conditions

As nonequilibrium systems, human beings are highly sensitive to stimuli. Early experiences can profoundly impact a life, creating vastly different outcomes. This occurrence, called *sensitivity to initial conditions*, is better known by its popular name, the *butterfly effect*. Coming from a paper *Predictability: Does the flap of a butterfly's wings in Brazil set off a tornado in Texas?*, the meteorologist Edward Lorenz (1972) demonstrated that even minor early alterations to a nonlinear system such as the weather can produce great changes over time. In human lives, we see its negative aspect when childhood abuse creates a life of emotional difficulties. Its positive aspect is evident in the far-from-equilibrium state of inspiration that begins a creative project and in the early creative trance that can start an adult career. E. B. White (1899–1985) decided to become a writer during a childhood creative trance. Held in rapt attention by a sheet of paper when he was age seven or eight, White (cited in Sweet, 2019, p. 1) stared at it "square in the eyes" and realized, "This is where I belong, this is it."

The Self-Organized Criticality, Punctuated Evolution, and the Creative Trance

Self-organization can occur on a spectrum from minor changes in a system to what may become global transformations. In nonequilibrium dissipative structures, where even small stimuli can produce large results, there are times when a system reaches a critical point and responds with a self-organization so strong that it produces a significant state change. Called a self-organized criticality, it appears to be intrinsic to dissipative systems (Bak et al., 1988; Bak, 1996).

Bak (1996) believes that large complex nonlinear systems like the brain evolve through these "flashing, intermittent bursts" of self-organized criticalities, rather than through gradual change. His theory of punctuated cognitive evolution has similarities with the paleobiological theory of punctuated equilibria (Gould & Eldredge, 1977), where slow gradual evolutionary change is punctuated by spurts of speciation. This theory postulates that the critical events of speciation, which generate distinctly new species, are what drive evolution forward. Human advancement through punctuated evolution becomes obvious when critical events, such as an illness or a trauma, impel us to alter our ways of living, thinking, and working (Zausner, 2016).

Bak (1996) sees the brain as a nonlinear system that changes through states of punctuated evolution. He finds that the brain not only has the capacity but also the *tendency* to self-organize into critical nonequilibrium states, such as flashes of insight, which promote cognitive advancement. Critical points are also inherent in the creative trance where decisions, changes, and new pathways form in response to a series of self-organized criticalities that punctuate the generation of a creative work. In mirroring a brain that advances through repeated self-organizations, the punctuated self-organization inherent in the creative process may also enhance our evolution and the evolution of the work. We appear to be primed for self-evolution by a brain and a creative trance that both impel us forward.

Self-Organized Criticalities and Avalanche Behavior

Self-organizing critical brain states may be modeled as avalanches of sand triggered by seemingly minor stimuli, such as thoughts or passing observations (Bak et al., 1988; Bak, 1996). Evidence of neural avalanche-type behavior has been found in networks of neurons, using EEG measurements (de Arcangelis et al., 2006). Associated with neural plasticity because these events can modify the circuitry between synapses, they may offer information about the processes of punctuated evolution in the brain.

In their neural criticality hypothesis, Hesse and Gross (2014) suggest that criticality may be an evolutionary trait fundamental to brain functioning because structures at critical points have optimum capabilities for memory and for information processing. Creative people may intuitively realize this in their creative trance because across domains they repeatedly push themselves toward critical points in their pursuit of excellence. If one aspect of work starts to come too easily, it may signal the time to start something new. Creative individuals are not only problem-solving people but problem-finding people. They look for challenges, which can lead to criticalities, spurring their work to grow and evolve.

Self-Organized Criticalities and the Pursuit of Excellence

Even when a criticality does not arise from within the work but is a trauma in life, creative people can turn it into a phase change for personal and professional growth (Zausner, 2016). After partial paralysis, almost total memory loss, and impaired vision from a head-on automobile accident, the visual artist Ginny Ruffner (b. 1952) reinvented herself and her work. Creativity with its creative trance is central to her. Self-described as a "lemon-to-lemonade type of person" (cited in Zausner, 2016, p. 29), Ruffner insisted, "It was as if life said to me, you want a challenge? Try this!"

There are also challenges we choose that may be modeled as continual criticalities, such as the sustained efforts necessary on the path to excellence. Research suggests that it takes approximately ten years or ten thousand hours of practice to achieve expertise in a field (Hayes, 2002; Vorwerg, 2019). In examining this length of time more closely, it appears to be structured by multiple criticalities.

According to the neural criticality hypothesis (Hesse & Gross, 2014), criticalities exist at the border between two qualitatively separate forms of behavior. This can be metaphorically modeled as a clarinetist reaching a breakthrough to a better level of performance and then using those increased skills to reach another breakthrough to a yet higher level of accomplishment. This sequence of states suggests a fractal pattern because they reoccur in a self-similar but not exact form as goals are met and then are continually elevated to achieve increasingly greater levels of success.

Self-Organized Criticalities: Catharsis and the Creative Trance

Deep emotional experiences, such as a profound insight or a catharsis, which is the release of intense constrained feelings, can be a self-organized criticality that structures a creative trance. Marcel Proust (1871–1922) wrote about his experience of catharsis in a novel, *The Remembrance of Things Past* (1913/2006). Feeling very depressed on a rainy gray day in winter, Proust's entire mood shifted to joy when he had a madeleine pastry with a cup of tea. Immediately, almost forgotten happy memories from childhood flooded his mind and he thought of his kind Aunt Leonie, who gave him tea-soaked Madeleines when he was a boy.

I have seen the flooding of cathartic memories produce a creative trance of emotional transformation in my therapy practice. One of my patients, a woman aged eighty-seven, had a cathartic experience when she spoke about her fears of being left behind. The woman lived with her son and daughter-in-law who were discussing their impending move to a different part of the city. Realizing my patient was very frightened; her son provided immediate assurance that she would be coming with them. Overwhelmed with feelings of relief and joy, my patient said it immediately triggered an earlier memory from over eighty years ago.

She was about age five then and just recovering from a severe case of diphtheria. Weak and unable to walk, she was put in a small chair in her bedroom while the whole family rushed around, packing for their move to a new house. When her older sister realized that the child was petrified of being left behind, she said, "Of course we are taking you with us!" In response, her distress turned to joy. Linking the two incidents, my patient's cathartic transformation from anxiety to security became a creative trance for her by producing a stronger sense of self and the confidence that she was part of a family. "Here I was," she said, "both times very weak and frail, thinking I might be abandoned, and yet so happy I was not going to be left behind."

Self-Organized Criticalities: Insight and the Creative Trance

Insight can also become a self-organized criticality leading to a profound cognitive shift (Gabora, 2017). This happened to the author and activist Helen Keller (1880–1968) when a childhood creative trance opened the door to increased communication. At the age of nineteen months, Keller (1996, p. 3) had a severe illness that her doctor called "an acute congestion of the stomach and brain." It took both Keller's hearing and her sight, leaving her in a dark silent world of very limited communication.

Everything changed at age six when Keller's teacher, Annie Sullivan, poured water on her hand while spelling the letters w-a-t-e-r on her palm. For the first time Keller associated the different pressures on her palm with letters that spelled out a word connected to the physical world. Describing her insight as a lightning bolt and an epiphany, it opened the door to verbal communication. Keller went on to earn a bachelor's degree from Harvard University, write books, and advocate for the rights of disabled people.

A Negative Self-Organized Criticality and the Creative Trance

Not all self-organizing criticalities are positive. The novelist Charles Dickens (1812–1870) had an extremely negative response to even the slightest odor from the glue that was used to paste labels (Ackerman, 1990). It brought back the devastating anguish Dickens felt as a child when he worked pasting labels onto bottles in a rat-infested factory. After his father was imprisoned for unpaid debts, Dickens was forced to leave school at age twelve to earn money for the family.

The conditions of his employment were so severe, that Dickens later reported, "No words can express the secret agony of my soul . . . the sense I had of being utterly neglected and hopeless; of the shame I felt in my position . . . My whole nature was penetrated with grief and humiliation" (cited in Tomalin, 2012, p. 25). As an adult, Dickens repeatedly used the effects of this trauma in his novels by alerting the public to the plight of disadvantaged children.

The Self-Organized Criticalities of Panic Attacks

Another experience suggesting the presence of a self-organized criticality is the panic attack, also known as panic disorder. Here, the initial state would be an elevated level of anxiety. The critical point is a stimulus, either consciously perceived such as a fear of crowds, or unconsciously received making the panic attack seem to arise "out of the blue." It is possible that the unconscious source of a panic attack may lie in the activity of the preconscious mind, that part of the unconscious that is closest to conscious awareness (Freud, 1963; Kihlstrom, 1987).

Contents of the preconscious are potentially available to the conscious mind and can theoretically direct both thought and behavior. The preconscious contains memories, and it is possible that the stimulus to panic may incite the dynamic of associative memory. By connecting disparate items, associative memory may correlate a present occurrence with past distress. Even though the activating stimulus may be a micro event, too small for conscious perception, it may still be registered by the continual monitoring of the unconscious mind.

Gabora and Kaufman (2010, p. 5) point out that "neurons are sensitive to *subsymbolic microfeatures* – primitive attributes of a stimulus, such as a sound of a particular pitch or a line of a particular orientation," and that this provides "an anatomical basis for self-triggered recall." Although they do not apply these dynamics to panic disorder, it is possible that the reception of a micro stimulus in the preconscious mind or at the liminal edge of preconscious to conscious awareness may be enough to start a cascade of events that form the self-organized criticality of a panic attack.

Panic Attacks and the Energy States of Nonlinear Dynamics

The panic phase is a time of extreme terror, dread, and discomfort. Symptoms of a panic attack may include palpitations, difficulty breathing, dizziness, shaking, trembling, tingling, body temperature changes, derealization, and depersonalization, along with a terrifying fear of dying, losing control, or losing sanity (World Health Association, 1992; American Psychiatric, 2013). Just as a small stimulus can have great effects on nonlinear systems, so can it generate an intense response in the nonlinear system of the mind.

Panic attacks tend to be recurrent, and their repetition without resolution may be described as a limit cycle in nonlinear dynamics (Zausner, 1999). In limit cycles there is a back-and-forth movement that never advances, like the swing of a pendulum. Limit cycles, with their cyclic attractors, have less energy than states of chaos. There appear to be four energy states described in chaos theory, each with a specific amount of energy and a type of movement. These four states, which are based on Conway's mathematical *Game of Life* with its computer-generated cellular automata (Waldrop, 1992), were categorized by Wolfram (1984) and then Langton (1992).

In the lowest energy state, Class I, there is a point attractor, with brief movement toward a point that ceases when the point is reached. Class II, a limit cycle with a cyclic attractor, has more energy but not enough to move forward out of its repetitive path. The increased energy of Class III with its strange attractor is a state of chaos, full of possibilities, where cells interact and combine into complex new formations. Class IV with more energy is over-energized and its cells form no lasting connections. It is a state of disorder with no definitive attractor, suggesting the extreme agitation and turmoil of panic without structure or resolution.

Turning Panic Attacks into a Creative Chaos

Panic attacks are uncomfortable, cyclical, and disorderly, yet they hold the potential for a strengthened sense of self and for a creative trance that generates works of art. The first and most obvious way to eliminate panic is to address the state of anxiety that is the prelude to its occurrence. Techniques such as relaxation, meditation, and acknowledging and expressing feelings can reduce anxiety levels and diminish the inclination to panic (Bourne, 2020). Also helpful is examining possible triggers, the circumstances of the panic attack, and the causes leading to a person's emotional state at the time.

If a panic attack does occur, there are ways that may turn the panic into a creative chaos. Models from nonlinear dynamics indicate that it is necessary both to add energy to the Class II limit cycle aspect of a panic attack, bringing it up to the Class III state of chaos, and to reduce the turmoil of over-active energies of the Class IV aspect. When controlled, the energy may contain a potential for productivity, like the creative chaos of Class III.

When a panic attack happens, the first steps are to name the occurrence a *panic attack* and then disengage from it by distracting yourself. Distractions end the panic attack by turning the mind to another subject or activity. Any distraction that engages the brain can be effective, ranging from redirecting thoughts to physical movements, such as cleaning or organizing, which take energy away from the panic and use it for a positive purpose.

Panic Attacks: Naming as Power and Rumpelstiltskin

Identifying the panic by naming it as a panic attack and not an impending demise, is an example of self-efficacy and produces a strengthened sense of self. It also adds energy to a system in the form of insight, lifting the panic attack from a limit cycle into a possible creative chaos of self-evolution. Naming creates distance by containing the emotional turmoil with a metaphorical strange attractor of identification. Recognizing the occurrence as a temporary non-life-threatening panic attack and not the prelude to annihilation enables disengagement, restores control, and makes the panic feel like a finite rather than a final event.

Naming as power has an archaic lineage. In ancient Egypt, the Goddess Isis made the Sun God Ra reveal his true name to her, thereby gaining power over him (Jung, 1976); and in the Judeo-Christian Bible (Genesis, 2:19), Adam is granted dominion over animals through naming them. In a European fairy tale (Grimm, 1972), a young Queen assumes power over an angry gnome by discovering that his name is *Rumpelstiltskin*. The Queen, psychologically symbolic of the rational mind, gains control over an angry gnome, symbolizing a negative eruption of the unconscious, analogous to the cause of a panic attack (Zausner, 1999).

Rumpelstiltskin reveals the enormous abilities of the unconscious mind by spinning straw into gold, but then tries to overpower the conscious mind by attempting to take away the Queen's infant child, symbolizing her new creative productivity. Finding and saying Rumpelstiltskin's name banishes the gnome forever and allows the Queen to keep her child. In parallel, finding and naming a previously hidden source of distress can stop a panic attack and inspire psychological healing and new creativity.

Panic Attacks and the Creative Trance in Poetry and Visual Art

Creative people have a history of turning panic into productivity by using the trauma as a recurrent theme in their work. This is apparent in the poet Emily Dickinson and the visual artist Edvard Munch. Both individuals had extreme panic in their lives and used its resulting distress as a repeated motif in their creative trance. Expressing trauma through creativity is a basis of the creative arts therapies and appears to have been therapeutic for both Dickinson and Munch.

In nonlinear dynamics, the expression and repetition of trauma in creative work suggests a fractal organization. The original trauma stands in a fractal relationship to the multiple instances it appears in the creative work. Its expression and repetition indicate an attempt at psychologically controlling the disturbance, encapsulating it to reduce the negative impact. Its dynamic encapsulation implies the psychological presence of a strange attractor that acknowledges the trauma yet creates boundaries for it in both art and life. An additional factor is the centering aspect of a creative trance, which directs attention to the work and away from the self.

Emily Dickinson: The Functions of Poetry and Panic

In January 1854, the poet Emily Dickinson (1830–1886) was at a meeting in church when she abruptly developed extreme anxiety, fear, and distressing physical symptoms that were consistent with a panic attack (McDermott, 2000; Archer, 2009). Although consciously realizing she had nothing to fear, Dickinson was overcome with a great terror, and described it as an overwhelming experience of chaos. The church aisles seemed to be visually distorted, and she was trembling. Although Dickinson became calmer as the church service progressed, she expressed enormous relief upon reaching her home.

A series of panic attacks followed, with symptoms that she later referred to as a chaos, leaving Dickinson severely agoraphobic as her life progressed. Yet her homebound existence provided the solitude that some creative people need to create (Kaufman & Gregoire, 2016). Dickinson, who wrote almost eighteen hundred poems and over a thousand letters, created poetry in response to trauma. Revealing in a letter, "I had a terror . . . and so I sing as the Boy does by the Burying Ground – because I am afraid" (cited in McDermott, 2000, p. 73). Another letter describes how her creative trance of writing calms the trembling of panic, "I felt a palsy here – the verses just relieve" (cited in Archer, 2009, p. 257).

An additional calming aspect may be the multiple mentions of death in her poems. This repetition to gain control of a fear may act as a metaphorical strange attractor encompassing and controlling the panic attack's greatest dread, that of annihilation. Yet Dickinson's panic appears to hold a secondary gain. Her anxiety may have functioned as the needed energy for a creative chaos, escaping the limitations imposed by a secluded existence. Dickinson alluded to this by writing (loc. 2209), "The stimulus there is in danger," and says (cited in Archer, 2009, p. 273), "My loss, by sickness -Was it Loss? Or that Ethereal Gain One earns by measuring the Grave – Then – measuring the Sun."

Edvard Munch: Anxiety and an Image of Panic Worldwide

The visual artist Edvard Munch (1863–1944) also transformed panic disorder into the deterministic chaos of a creative trance. He revealed, "Without illness and anxiety, I would have been a rudderless ship" (cited in Potter, 2011, p. 573). Extremely anxious and frightened of heights and open spaces, Munch had what is probably the most famous panic attack in the world when he was left alone on a bridge in Oslo overlooking the fjord.

He depicted the event in his 1893 painting *The Scream*, which has since become an international icon. The image shows an ageless nongendered person turning away in fear from a railing overlooking water and land far below. The figure, in severe distress with wide-open eyes and mouth, is holding its head with its hands on either side, in a way that magnifies the experience of terror. Munch made multiple paintings and prints of *The Scream*, presumably to gain psychological control over his distress.

The effort to confront trauma through its repetition in works of art, suggests the presence of a metaphorical strange attractor containing the anxiety and presenting it in a more manageable form. The created images then stand in a fractal relationship to the artist's experience and to each other. They also stand in a fractal relationship to the many images of *The Scream* in popular culture. Appearing on items including clothing, coffee mugs, and pillows, people around the world see in Munch's work a fractal reflection of their own anxiety. Then in an audience creative trance, the humor with which the images are presented may possibly allow these viewers to lessen the stress of their own experience.

Creativity and the Creative Trance in a Nonlinear World

Creativity is like swimming through constantly moving waters filled with unknown currents and limitless surprises. Yet continued exposure to this chaos strengthens the creative person and deepens the creative trance, making the work stronger, more unique, and more profound. The interaction within and between nonlinear systems is continuous and global, making us constantly evolving emergent phenomena in a continuously evolving emergent world.

CHAPTER 8

Dyslexia, Attention-Deficit Disorder, and the Creative Trance

A wounded deer leaps highest

Emily Dickinson

You can't use up creativity. The more you use, the more you have

Maya Angelou

Whatever affects the brain structures the creative trance. What we view as imperfections may be alternate pathways to achievement. None of us is perfect and perfection, as Jung (1978) points out, is an abstract and unattainable goal. Instead, he advises to access our inner dynamic wholeness, the aspect that transcends perfection and fuels self-evolution. The creative people in this chapter use neural challenges to access their wholeness, and this in turn, drives and shapes their creative trance. Although there are many types of neural challenges, this chapter will focus on two of the most common, dyslexia and attention-deficit disorder, now known as ADHD (attention deficit hyperactivity disorder). What makes life most difficult can also inspire strength and motivation.

Neural Challenges and the Creative Trance

The neural challenges of learning disorders may more accurately be viewed as learning differences. Then instead of impediments, they can be appreciated as opportunities to construct new pathways into a creative trance. There are many conditions considered to be learning disorders, but this chapter will concentrate on dyslexia. I have dyslexia and it affects my work and my life. Sometimes people with severe learning differences, like Leonardo da Vinci (1452–1519), who appears to have had dyslexia and the mixed type of ADHD, are labeled as unintelligent and told they would never be successful (Zausner, 2016). Yet despite multiple condemnations that left a deep legacy of emotional scars, Leonardo created works of genius across multiple domains.

Dyslexia

Dyslexia is usually an inherited condition, identified by difficulties in reading, spelling, and writing in people with satisfactory intelligence, eyesight, and educational opportunities (Zausner, 2016). Some individuals with dyslexia may reverse letters or numbers, have problems recognizing letters, relating words to their sounds, or they may see only part of a word or a group of numbers. Dyslexic difficulties are neurological, originating from brain abnormalities in regions including the corpus callosum, the cerebellum, and the left posterior cortex, all of which generate different types of learning problems (Beaton, 2004). In primary dyslexia, the problems are lifelong, while in developmental dyslexia, they lessen with maturity.

Currently a recognized learning disorder, dyslexia is treated by educational programs that can distinguish learning difficulties from evidence of diminished intellectual capacities. By acknowledging that people with dyslexia may have normal and in certain cases superior intelligence, they aim to reverse former assumptions that considered people with dyslexia as deficient. This inaccurate labeling in the past often left people with a profound loss of self-esteem, yet it is now known that dyslexic individuals can be brilliant. Some widely accomplished creative people with dyslexia include Albert Einstein, Thomas Alva Edison, Agatha Christie, William Butler Yeats, Leonardo da Vinci, Pablo Picasso, and Rosa Bonheur (Aaron et al., 1988; West, 1997; Zausner, 2016).

Dyslexia, the Brain, Visualization, and Science

There are anatomical markers in the brains of people with developmental dyslexia. Galaburda (1983, 1989) found they had more hemispheric symmetry with less neural pruning, and while the brains showed malformations in the perisylvian regions of the cerebral cortex relevant to language there was increased right hemisphere development compared to non-dyslexic individuals. Galaburda suggests that the more developed right hemispheric neural connections may account for the disproportionately greater evidence of creativity in the dyslexic population. It is also possible that this right hemispheric advantage may enable an enhanced capacity for visualization, which is a primary aspect of the creative trance.

West (1997) believes that people with dyslexia tend to be visual thinkers. He cites the Nobel Prize–winning immunologist Baruj Benacerraf (1920–2011), who found his ability to visualize objects in three-dimensional space was a great advantage in scientific research. Benacerraf was an extremely dyslexic child able to read only one word at a time. He also appeared to have dysgraphia, a neurological disorder identified by writing problems such as poor spelling and distorted or incorrect letters. Benacerraf said he found a way to read through hard work and will power, and that later, computers helped his spelling and handwriting difficulties.

Three other Nobel Laureates who were visual thinkers with language difficulties are the theoretical physicists Albert Einstein (1879–1955), Richard Feynman (1918–1988), and Niels Bohr (1885–1962). As a child, Bohr often "wrote incorrectly" with poor spelling and handwriting, and as an adult he preferred to dictate his writing (Pais, 1991, p. 49). Neither Einstein nor Feynman spoke until they were age three. Pinker (1999) suggests this language delay, which can occur in people with exceptional mathematical abilities, may be the result of different brain regions competing for space in the developing cerebral cortex. Sowell (2020, p. 89) notes that children with high intelligence may not only begin talking later but may also have what is known as "The pathology of superiority," which includes a greater incidence of myopia, immune disorders, and allergies, even though their overall health tends to be better than that of the general population.

When Dyslexia Influences the Choice of Profession

Dyslexia can affect a creative trance by influencing the choice of profession. Difficulties in reading or recognizing numbers may cause people to seek careers that focus less on words or numbers. My first choice of career would have been physics or mathematics, but I am dyslexic and often cannot see all the numbers in an equation. Writing is also difficult for me; I write very slowly and make many revisions. For the first part of my life, until I became a psychologist, I concentrated on visual art and continue to be a visual artist.

Dean Moss (b. 1954), an interdisciplinary choreographer and video artist with dyslexia, initially wanted to be an astronaut. Yet when he applied to the Naval Academy, they told him to return to school for a year to raise his "terrible English scores" (Moss & Lee, 2012, p. 59). While taking humanities courses at a community college, Moss discovered dance classes and they opened the world of choreography to him. Describing his joy as a creative trance response to the success of one of his multimedia dance performances, Moss (p. 63) called it a "constant tide of bliss that keeps sweeping over. It's just breathtaking."

Schnitt (1990), who finds a high incidence of dyslexia among dancers, suggests there may be a correlation between the learning disorder and an enhanced kinesthetic sense. While there have been studies linking dyslexia with possible deficits in motor control (Fawcett & Nicolson, 1995; Ramus et al., 2003), the opposite also appears to be true.

Reading can generate a creative trance in childhood that begins the trajectory to an adult career. While reading may be an impediment for a dyslexic child, if the book is translated into visual media, it may have the same effect. The oceanographer Robert Ballard (b. 1942) says, "I'm dyslexic, and that I learn differently. I didn't read *Twenty Thousand Leagues Under the Sea*; I watched the movie produced by Disney" (cited in Hardingham-Gill, 2021, online). It became an inspiration for Ballard, who went on to discover underwater hydrothermal vent ecosystems and find the submerged *Titanic*.

Dyslexia and Visual Artists

Research indicating a heightened capacity for manual dexterity in people with dyslexia (West, 1997) may explain their noticeable presence in the visual arts. Eminent artists with dyslexia include Leonardo da Vinci (1452–1519), Pablo Picasso (1881–1973), August Rodin (1840–1917), Rosa Bonheur (1822–1899), and Robert Rauschenberg (1925–2008) (Zausner, 2016). A primary reason for choosing visual art was their extreme difficulty in reading. As Rauschenberg admitted, "Probably the only reason that I'm a painter is because I couldn't read" (cited in McKendry, 1976, p. 34). Bonheur and Picasso had artist fathers who trained them, and they may have become artists even without learning disorders. Yet Picasso's father still feared that his young son might grow up to be nearly illiterate.

Exchanging the stress of letters for the creative trance of making visual art is not only a relief, but it can also generate a transcendent experience. The sculptor August Rodin (1840–1917) had dyslexia, which prevented him from becoming the professional or civil servant his parents wanted him to be (Champigneulle, 1967). Instead, he went to art school. Toward the beginning of classes, when Rodin opened the door to a sculpture studio, he recalled (cited in Champigneulle, 1967, p. 14), "I saw clay for the first time, and I felt as if I were ascending into heaven."

Dyslexia, Trauma, and the Creative Trance

A very difficult aspect of dyslexia is the repeated trauma it may cause a child who is struggling to read. Recurrent failures can generate lifelong scars, leading to a profound loss of self-esteem. The inability with words may escalate into a negative self-identity as it did with Leonardo da Vinci (1970a, p. 14), who called himself a *homo sanza lettere* (a man without letters). Rosa Bonheur remembered that in her childhood, "Beads of sweat would collect on my forehead while my mother wore herself out trying to drum the alphabet into my head" (cited in Klumpke, 1997, p. 87).

Recalling his distress in school, Robert Rauschenberg (cited in Mattison, 2003, p. 37) said, "I grew up being reassured every day that I was inferior." Yet the dyslexia that caused him distress when he saw letters backward in school became an asset in his creative trance. During printmaking the created image is reversed when printed, but Rauschenberg, who was able to see images reversed, did not have to make multiple trial proofs before the final print, as most artists do. He explained (cited in McKendry, 2003, p. 34), "I already see things backwards! You see, in printmaking everything comes out backwards so printing is an absolute natural for me." Seeing upside down and backward also influenced Rauschenberg's paintings because he would render some of his images that way. In response, he drew critical praise for incorporating multiple perspectives in his work (Mattison, 2003).

Dyslexia and the Musical Creative Trance

A research study by Nelson and Hourigan (2016) focusing on five nationally recognized musicians who have dyslexia discloses similarities to creative people with dyslexia in other domains. All five musicians (their identities were withheld) had difficulties reading text and three could not read music. This led to problems with schoolwork, and the resulting trauma caused poor self-esteem. Yet the negative self-image left by academic courses was countered by success in music. As one of the musicians said, "Music was the healthiest thing that happened to me" (p. 58). Their creative trance of music also became a creative trance of healing. Like dance for the choreographer Dean Moss, and visual art for the artists discussed earlier, music became a domain in which they could excel.

Dyslexia appears to enhance the capacity for visualization or otherwise experiencing a creative work in the mind (West, 1997). As part of the musicians' creative trance, they could hear music. One of the participants believed that his dyslexia gave him (p. 58) "the ability to hear an original song mentally as if a recording were playing. This mental hearing would include the complete orchestration." The musicians could visualize easily and two of them mentioned the ability to see things from multiple points of view, reminiscent of the capacity for multiple perspectives in Rauschenberg's paintings.

The three musicians who were unable to read musical notation found other ways to learn and remember music. They listened to recordings of the scores they were to play, visually memorized finger movements needed to make the music, and focused on technology, using instruments connected to a computer or other digital interface and computer programs that completely bypassed musical notation. Their multisensory approach to music appears to have similarities with the multimedia approach that Dean Moss takes for choreography. Overy (2000, 2003) advocates music lessons for dyslexic children because of their potential to provide a multisensory approach to learning. She suggests that in dyslexia there are deficits in temporal processing, a type of neurological timing, and believes that music training, which requires accurate timing, may have the capacity to improve literacy skills.

Eminent Authors with Dyslexia and the Writer's Creative Trance

Difficulties from dyslexia do not always influence the choice of profession. While it may sound paradoxical, there are eminent authors with dyslexia, including Agatha Christie (1890–1976), F. Scott Fitzgerald (1896–1940), Jules Verne (1828–1905), and William Butler Yeats (1865–1939) (Regents of the University of Michigan, 2020). Some of these individuals with dyslexia also had dysgraphia, such as the world's bestselling novelist, Agatha Christie (2010, p. 55), who said that "both writing and spelling were a pain to me." Later in life, Christie experimented with dictation but returned to typing and writing her manuscripts, because dictation negatively altered her creative trance. She found it made her language too verbose and believed that an "economy of wording ... is particularly necessary in detective stories" (p. 341).

Yet why would people with language problems struggle to create in a domain where they are neurologically challenged? The writer Paul Ford (b. 1944) believes dyslexia makes him a better writer because he is a slow reader. Ford says (cited in Burns, 2008, p. 201) that "being slow made me pore over sentences and to be receptive to ... the 'poetical' aspects of language." Another reason appears to be a profound urge for self-expression through verbal means. Writers are our storytellers; it is part of their self-identity, their ground of being. Central to human civilization, storytelling is prized across cultures. Deriving from an ancient lineage, possibly concurrent with the acquisition of verbal language, storytelling creates a creative trance in the teller and an audience creative trance in the listener. Ford speaks about this set of creative trances, saying that reading stories brought completion to incomplete aspects of his life, and that he wants to do this for others.

Humans have been telling stories for thousands of years, but widespread literacy is only a recent phenomenon. When most humans could neither read nor write, learning disorders were generally unrecognized (Zausner, 2016) and storytellers with dyslexia might not have been aware of it. As a primary transmission of culture, words are central to society. This may be why, despite generations of dyslexia, the genetics for storytelling have been preserved throughout millennia. The success of its heritability becomes apparent when the talent appears in families. Agatha Christie's mother and sister were also storytellers (Christie, 2010, 2020).

Attention Deficit/Hyperactivity Disorder and the Brain

ADHD, attention deficit hyperactivity disorder, formerly known as attention-deficit disorder (ADD), is a behavioral syndrome that usually begins in childhood (Cortese et al., 2012; American Psychiatric Association, 2013; Volkow & Swanson, 2013; Thomas et al., 2015). Appearing in up to 7.2 percent of children worldwide, it can be inherited or acquired, and may continue into adulthood for up to 65 percent of the individuals. ADHD, which is associated with disorganization, impulsivity, and difficulty in completing projects, presents with either symptoms of excessive motor behavior, such as restlessness, fidgeting, excessive talking, and interrupting, or with symptoms of inattentive behavior, such as distractibility, mind wandering, inattention, and forgetfulness, or a combination of both aspects. For some individuals, ADHD may affect their schoolwork, employment, and social interactions.

Brain scans of people with ADHD show the involvement of multiple regions. Volkow and Swanson (2013) find that while there is less activity in the brain networks dedicated to attention and executive function, there is increased activation of the default mode network with its capacity for mind wandering and its focus on the inner states of the self. Stefanatos and Wasserstein (2001) suggest ADHD may be a spectrum of disorders involving right hemisphere compromise in the frontal and parietal regions. They connect the impulsive hyperactive subtype of ADHD with deficiencies in the anterior systems of the right hemisphere and the inattentive type with problems in posterior functioning.

The syndrome appears to alter with age because adults with ADHD tend to retain symptoms of inattention but have fewer aspects of hyperactivity (Volkow & Swanson, 2013). We see this in brain scans where children with ADHD have increased activation of the somatomotor networks while adults do not. Both children and adults with ADHD show lower activation in the frontoparietal network, which is associated with executive function, including self-regulation. Yet they have higher activation in areas such as the default network, indicating a focus on the inner rather than the outside world. Adults with ADHD also had increased activation of the visual network, which may indicate a greater propensity for visualization. Higher activity in the default and visual networks suggests an aptitude to daydream, to visualize, and to enter a creative trance more easily.

Eminent People with Attention Deficit/Hyperactivity Disorder

There are eminent people across domains whose ADHD structured their creative trance. The inventor Thomas Alva Edison (1847–1931) appeared to benefit from his combined form of ADHD, using the reveries for creativity and the active aspect in his life as an entrepreneur. In childhood, Edison had evidence of dysgraphia with difficulties in punctuation, capitalization, spelling, and grammar, which placed him bottom in his class (Hallowell & Ratey, 1994; West, 1997). Yet it was the mind-wandering of ADHD that stopped his formal education. Edison's teacher called him "addled" and expelled the boy in three months (Mould, 2016, p. 500). Afterward, he was homeschooled by his mother and read extensively on his own. Edison, who only slept four to five hours a night, liked to nap and napping was a vehicle for his creative trance. In that half-waking hypnagogic state before sleep (Krippner, 1999a), creative ideas would drift into his consciousness.

The poet Robert Frost (1874–1963), who is presumed to have had ADHD, was also expelled from school for excessive daydreaming; and the architect Frank Lloyd Wright (1867–1959) daydreamed so deeply in childhood because of ADHD that it was hard to wake him (Cramond, 1994). The physicist Albert Einstein (1879–1955) also appears to have had ADHD (Hallowell & Ratey, 1994). A shy, withdrawn, and lonely child with hesitant speech, Einstein was thought to be dull at home and at school (Goertzel & Goertzel, 1962, p. 248). A teacher once told his parents that Einstein was "mentally slow, unsociable, and adrift forever in his foolish dreams." One of Einstein's daydreams at age sixteen (Weinstein, 2017) was the visualization of himself riding a light beam that became a foundation for the theory of special relativity.

With its similarities to creative thinking (Cramond, 1994; Zausner, 2016), ADHD appears to be widespread in the creative population. The list of famous people who reportedly had ADHD is quite long and includes the composer Amadeus Mozart, (1756–1791), the actors Whoopi Goldberg (b. 1955), Robin Williams (1951–2014), Dustin Hoffman (b. 1937), and Lindsay Wagner (b. 1949) (Hallowell & Ratey, 1994; Schmitt & Falkai, 2014). Although the artist Walt Disney (1901–1966) is often cited as having ADHD, his diagnosis is uncertain. It is possible that exhaustion from getting up at 3:30 a.m. for a paper route before school kept Disney from staying alert during class (Zausner, 2016). The baseball player Andres Torres is very public about having ADHD and his struggle to stay focused in sports. After getting treatment for his condition, Torres became a spokesperson for ADHD awareness in the film about his life, *Gigante: A Documentary* (NYU Langone Health, 2012).

How ADHD Structures the Creative Trance: States of Reverie and Fleeting Attention

When characteristics of ADHD are similar to aspects of the creative process, they appear to promote creativity (Cramond, 1994; Zausner, 2016) and structure a creative trance. A very strong connection is the link between the inattentive daydreaming aspect of ADHD and the altered state of a creative trance. Inattention and daydreaming may contain the visualizations necessary to inspire and complete a creative project. In the reveries of ADHD, there is a heightened activation of the default mode network allowing access to inner states of mind and an increased proximity to the creativity of the unconscious.

Inner states of reverie accessed in a creative trance provide the mental time and space to work on ideas before translating them into physical reality. Mozart, who had ADHD (Schmitt & Falkai, 2014), could compose entire symphonies in his mind before committing them to paper (Mozart, 1985), and the architect Frank Lloyd Wright visualized his projects in such detail that he needed very few preliminary drawings (Currey, 2014). Yet, these creative benefits can arise only if a person is not overwhelmed by severe ADHD where rapid thoughts can impede creativity and daydreams may remain unrealized in the physical world.

The changing focus of attention in ADHD can also assist creativity because it permits and encourages new ideas to come into conscious awareness. By keeping the mind available to many possibilities, it creates multiple options in the creative process. This psychological openness is an example of divergent thinking. White and Shah (2006) found that adults with ADHD outperformed those without ADHD on divergent thinking but did less well on convergent thinking. The creative process is often a combination of both, with convergent thinking providing the logic and structure. Yet it is divergent thinking that has the potential to bring civilization forward by generating new insights through the creativity of an active imagination.

How ADHD Structures the Creative Trance: Hyperfocus

It may sound paradoxical, but ADHD, a syndrome characterized by fleeting attention, also contains the capability for highly focused attention. In my anecdotal experience with creative individuals, this aspect of ADHD generates the most positive response because it aids accomplishment. It helps them get their work done. Popularly called *hyperfocus*, the capacity for extended episodes of concentration is not yet a diagnostic criterion for ADHD. While for some people hyperfocus can be a treasured experience that structures a creative trance, for others it can be negative when it impedes the capacity to shift focus (Brown, 2005).

In their research on adult ADHD, Hupfeld, Abagis, and Shah (2018) note that aspects of hyperfocus can include a heightened focus of attention, a sense of timelessness, engagement in a task, and an inward concentration turned away from the outside world. They find hyperfocus to be like the experience of flow (Csikszentmihalyi, 1990, 1996), but more immersive, and suggest it be considered a type of deep flow.

Yet the aspects of hyperfocus they cite have congruence with the state of a deep creative trance. Chapter 1 of this book presents three depths of a creative trance, light, medium, and deep, and compares the light creative trance with Csikszentmihalyi's concept of flow, where environmental sounds diminish with attention to a task. In the deepest creative trance, environmental distractions completely disappear, and time and space may seem nonexistent. It is possible that for some individuals, this deepest state of creative trance may also include an experience of hyperfocus.

How ADHD Structures the Creative Trance: Low Brain Arousal and Ambient Sound

Another aspect of ADHD that can affect the creative trance is the state of brain arousal. Individuals with ADHD tend to have lower and less stable brain arousal than the general population (Strauss et al., 2018). A cause might be either altered organization located primarily in the frontal regions of the brain (Loo et al., 2009), or possibly disruptions in the right hemisphere parietal regions (Stefanatos & Wasserstein, 2001). An ongoing state of hypoarousal in ADHD can create a need for heightened cortical activity to sustain attention (Loo et al., 2009; Mayer et al., 2016). This may be why some creative individuals with ADHD use background sound to facilitate their creative trance (Zausner, 2016).

Soderlund, Sikstrom, and Smart (2007) suggest that the use of an optimal level and type of sound can create a stochastic resonance, an occurrence of noise positively altering the behavior of a system. An example of this may be when external sound enhances the performance of some people with ADHD. Environmental noise comes into the neural system through sensory perception and becomes internal noise where it may compensate for the reduced brain arousal and low dopamine production in ADHD. Working with a background sound of either music or words to stimulate creative production is a widespread practice in the visual arts with historical roots (Zausner, 2016). In his writing on painting (1989, p. 39), Leonardo da Vinci says that while working, an artist "enjoys the accompaniment of music or the company of the authors of various fine works that can be heard with great pleasure."

As a visual artist with the mixed form of ADHD, I have used either music or words as a background screen when I paint. Initially, they energize me but then comes an experience of deep silence. Perhaps like the principle of destructive interference in physics, when waves cancel each other out, so the background sound and my internally perceived sound seem to nullify each other into silence. The work always moves forward in that extremely quiet time, the absolute best time to paint.

Leonardo da Vinci: Dyslexia, Dysgraphia, ADHD, and the World-Altering Creative Trance

The multiple challenges of Leonardo da Vinci (1452–1519) structured his creative trance and altered the course of Western culture. Leonardo, whose work ushered in the High Renaissance in visual art (Hartt, 1987), was a writer, painter, inventor, astronomer, engineer, mathematician, geologist, geographer, philosopher, city planner, architect, physicist, biologist, anatomist, botanist, musician, and a person with challenges.

Leonardo appears to have had dyslexia, dysgraphia, and both subtypes of ADHD, the daydreaming inattention and the restless impulsivity (Zausner, 2016). All these conditions were fundamental to his work.

When dyslexia and dysgraphia closed the doors to higher education, Leonardo relied on his own originality and became an astute observer of the natural world. While the behavioral syndrome ADHD led Leonardo to impulsivity, its divergent thinking and resulting inspirations enabled him to create works of genius. Using the deep reveries of ADHD for intensive visualization, he designed machines that worked perfectly five hundred years later when they were built from his drawings.

Leonardo da Vinci: Dyslexia and Dysgraphia

Leonardo, who called himself a *homo sanza lettere* (a man without letters), was painfully aware of his problems with written language (1970a, pp. 14–15). He stated, "They will say that I, having no literary skill, cannot properly express that which I desire to treat." Realizing that he wrote from right to left with reversed letters in a mirror script, it is now believed that Leonardo dictated all his business communication to Francesco Melzi, his well-educated and devoted pupil (Bambach, 2003b; Vecce, 2003). Melzi, who wrote with standard letters in the left to right format, also combined Leonardo's various pieces of writing into notebooks after the painter's death. It is Leonardo's mirror script with its reversed letters and numerous unusual misspellings that provides an intimation of his dyslexia and dysgraphia.

When Leonardo attempts to copy standard script into his notes, his handwriting appears to be strained and he still unintentionally reverses letters and numbers (Bambach, 2003). Like other individuals with dyslexia, who write in mirror script (Rawson, 1982), it may have been a more comfortable form of self-expression for Leonardo, allowing his ideas to flow unimpeded in a writer's creative trance. Leonardo's spelling appears to be phonological, by sound. Yet his numerous, unusual, and inconsistent errors, such as consonant doubling, splitting, or blending words, and letter substitutions, are not made by the general public and suggest a diagnosis of surface dysgraphia and developmental dyslexia (Sartori, 1987; Aaron et al., 1988; West, 1992). Leonardo also had problems with syntax, punctuation, and did not employ apostrophes or accent marks.

Aaron, Phillips, and Larsen (1988) believe Leonardo had difficulties reading because he appeared to process a word as a unit, rather than a compilation of sequential letters. In addition, they offer neurological evidence for developmental dyslexia, citing the stroke Leonardo had at age sixty-seven. Despite paralyzing his right arm, it did not affect his speech, as it would have done with most people suffering left hemisphere damage. Instead, they note that individuals with developmental dyslexia tend to have incomplete cerebral lateralization, resulting in a more diffuse cerebral organization with speech areas across both hemispheres.

Leonardo's dyslexia also appears to be developmental because as an adult he had a collection of books, and the Renaissance art historian Giorgio Vasari (1996) says that he was always seeking knowledge and read extensively. Like many people with dyslexia (Bowman & Culotta, 2010), it was difficult for Leonardo to learn a second language, although he tried to learn Latin in childhood and again as an adult (Vecce, 2003). In the Italian Renaissance, all higher education was given in Latin, and so the doors to a university education remained closed to him.

Leonardo da Vinci and the High Renaissance in Italian Art

Instead, Leonardo went to an abbaco, a school for future merchants. His father, Ser Piero da Vinci, an educated notary, which in the Renaissance was similar to a lawyer, then realized an art education would be more suited to his son's talents. He apprenticed Leonardo, at approximately age seventeen, to the very successful visual artist Andrea del Verrocchio (1435–1488) (Vasari, 1996; Dunkerton, 2011). In this busy Florentine workshop, which produced three-dimensional works as well as paintings, instruction was verbal, not written, and presented in Italian. Here, Leonardo soon surpassed his master, which, Vasari said, greatly distressed the elder Verrocchio. Yet, as Leonardo later wrote (1970a, p. 250), "He is a poor disciple who does not excel his master."

In Verrocchio's studio, Leonardo worked on *Baptism of Christ* c. 1470–1475, now in the Uffizi Galleries (2020). It shows evidence of his hand in the background landscape and in aspects of the image of Jesus, but most completely in the little angel turning around in the left foreground. Unlike the greater part of the painting, which is painted in a stiff linear style of the earlier Renaissance, Leonardo's image is markedly different. Simultaneously naturalistic and ethereal with subtle shading in the face and garments, it has intimations of movement. Leonardo was only in his twenties when he painted the small figure with its naturalism and grace. Yet his creative trance was one of constant innovation, and here it brought in a completely new era, the High Renaissance in Italian art.

Leonardo da Vinci and the Observer's Creative Trance

Even the great variety of artistic production in Verrocchio's workshop was not enough for Leonardo's constantly searching, creative, and scientific mind. He was a polymath, a person with wide-ranging interests and competencies. Denied the socially approved university credentials, and unable to quote from Latin texts like academic scholars, Leonardo defiantly carved a new direction for himself. Insisting that to quote from books is like wearing the literary garments of others, he says (Da Vinci, 1970a, p. 15), "though I may not, like them, be able to quote other authors, I shall rely on that which is much greater and more worthy: experience." Believing that (Da Vinci, 2005, p. 300) "all our knowledge has its origin in our perceptions," Leonardo used his creative trance of observation to become one of the greatest viewers in history.

The observer's trance is a creative experience because the brain is always forming new connections to stimuli impinging upon the senses. Leonardo believes observation must be continual and dismisses painters who walk only for relaxation without studying their surroundings. Instead, he states, "The mind of a painter must resemble a mirror, which always takes the color of the object it reflects and is completely occupied by the images of as many objects as are in front of it" (Da Vinci, 2005, p. 11). Yet his mirror has consciousness and a hierarchical nature.

While Leonardo instructs painters to retain images and facts in the mind, he advises them to be fully conscious of their existence, separating and retaining only those of greater value. Leonardo did not just observe the natural world, he analyzed his findings, illustrated them, and wrote his conclusions on thousands of pieces of paper that were later gathered as a compendium into the notebooks we have of his work (Da Vinci, 1970 a,b). Unfortunately, over the centuries many of his manuscripts were lost.

The Observer's Creative Trance as Inspiration for Originality

Using his creative trance of observation, Leonardo made astounding discoveries about the natural world that were often out of accordance with the knowledge of his time (Da Vinci, 1970a, 1970b, 1983). By studying striated rocks, Leonardo realized they were the result of successive geologic events. He also understood that the fossils of marine life found high in the mountains indicated the region was once at the bottom of a deep sea. By examining cracks in a wall, Leonardo uncovered the structural defects of a building.

His visual investigations included detailed illustrations of botany, landscapes, animals, physics, hydraulics, and astronomy, among other subjects. Leonardo's perceptions are so accurate that his drawings of turbulent water have been used in contemporary science to illustrate the fractal aspects of chaos theory (Mandelbrot, 1983). Leonardo was also a great anatomist, who dissected over thirty corpses and influenced modern medicine (Crowe & Wells, 2004; Bhattacharya & Neela, 2006). As Freud said (1989, p. 82), "He was like a man who had awoken too early in the darkness, while everyone else was still asleep."

Insisting that his "works are the issue of pure and simple experience" (1970a, p. 15), Leonardo codified his observations on perspective, color, proportions, light, and shade into instructions for visual artists. He was a strong proponent of reveries as a stimulus to creativity (p. 254), and suggests that artists enter a trance state through focused observation. Calling it "A way of developing and arousing the mind to various inventions," Leonardo recommends staring intensely at a wall with stains or stones. Eventually, he says, they will begin to resemble landscapes, battle scenes, costumes, and strange faces, all of which may be useful for visual art. Leonardo's method of visual associations, now considered to be a stream of consciousness connections, is regarded as a breakthrough in Renaissance creative thinking (Bambach, 2003a).

Leonardo da Vinci, ADHD, and the Creative Trance

Leonardo appears to have the mixed type of ADHD, with both the impulsivity and the daydreaming. According to Vasari (1996, pp. 625–626), Leonardo was a restless, impatient child in school who "didn't stay with any subject very long and asked so many questions that he bewildered his teacher." As an adult, he had erratic and unpredictable behavior. Although Leonardo moved his home multiple times, there were hours when he would be lost in thought, and he was widely known for leaving projects unfinished. Yet Vasari acknowledges that, throughout his life, Leonardo was constantly drawing and that he was always thinking.

Leonardo exemplifies what Cramond (1994) says are two types of ADHD restlessness in a creative person. There is the restlessness that keeps him from finishing his larger works and the restlessness that drives his production and they both structure his creative trance. Although Leonardo completed only fifteen paintings and none of his sculptures, he made over four thousand drawings, a number four times greater than anyone else of that era (Bambach, 2003a). The shorter time span necessary to make a drawing is more comfortable for a person with ADHD like Leonardo than the months or years needed to complete an oil painting or sculpture in the meticulous style of Renaissance art. As short-term projects, drawings provide the variety, speed, and novelty that match the attention span of a person with ADHD, and Leonardo drew quickly. The art historian Carmen Bambach (2003) calls the freshness in Leonardo's drawings a great innovation in Renaissance art.

ADHD also structures Leonardo's creative trance in writing, painting, and inventing. In his notebooks, Leonardo (1970a,b) writes briefly on many subjects in a succinct style that focuses on the important information and leaves out extraneous material. The daydreaming aspect of ADHD, so crucial for Leonardo's creativity, was a great aggravation to his patrons. When Leonardo was working on the mural of *The Last Supper*, for the Dominican monastery in Milan, he could be lost in thought for half a day. Seeing this, the Prior of the monastery accused him of doing nothing and complained to Ludovico Sforza, the Duke of Milan (Vasari, 1996).

In response, Leonardo insisted that the mind must first imagine what the hands will later create. He was a visual thinker with an imagination capable of rotating three-dimensional objects in his mind and drawing them from different angles (West, 1992). Leonardo visualized his inventions, such as a helicopter, a parachute, a bicycle, a human-powered glider, a spring-powered car, and a diving apparatus, so accurately and drew them so clearly that centuries later they could be completely constructed from his drawings.

Leonardo da Vinci, Tangential Thinking, Inspiration, and the Creative Trance

In addition to divergent and convergent thinking, I suggest there is also tangential thinking, which may occur in a person with ADHD. Tangential thinking is a type of inspiration that can happen during a creative trance when the project in progress acts as a stimulus to a new aspect of its own creativity or an entirely different creative endeavor. Although similar to impulsivity and distractibility, because it veers suddenly from one topic to another, tangential thinking is also very different because its purposeful interruption leads to increased creativity.

Tangential thinking is not like the thought disturbance of tangentiality (APA, 2020), where a person continually digresses to extraneous subject matter, never reaching a conclusion. It also differs from de Bono's (1990) concept of lateral thinking, which is a deliberate conscious method of problem-solving that uses logic to change from an existing pattern to a new one. Instead, tangential thinking is an impulsive diversion from a current line of creative thought to a new one. Sometimes tangential thinking can lead to a trail of associations going nowhere, but at other times, it brings flashes of insight and completely new work. Tangential thinking, which structures a creative trance, can be a common occurrence in individuals with ADHD like Leonardo (Zausner, 2016).

Yet not everyone admired Leonardo's tangential thinking, because it could bring inspirations out of order, interrupting the linear sequence of a project. When Leonardo received a painting commission from Pope Leo X, he became so focused on the varnish he would use on the finished work that he made the varnish before the painting (Vasari, 1996). The Pope was furious, saying the artist would never be a success, and gave him no more commissions. Yet for Leonardo, tangential thinking was a type of inspiration and a stimulus to invention. It is evident in his anatomical drawings of a hand, where he impulsively stops and makes a note to himself that he should write a book about the mechanics of movement in human and nonhuman animals (Keele, 1984). Leonardo's tangential thinking that arises in one subject inspires him to work in another, creating connections across disciplines and leading to works of genius in multiple domains.

Leonardo da Vinci: Depression, Anxiety, Self-Image, and Resilience

Included with his brilliant observations and analyses, Leonardo's notebooks also contain hints of an underlying depression, an ongoing lack of self-esteem, and anxiety that he is outside accepted social norms. Leonardo voices these concerns in the introduction to his notebook (1970a, p. 13), where he worries that those who came before him studied everything that was useful, leaving him only their "despised and rejected merchandise," their leftovers of lesser value. Leonardo believes he will not be able to distribute his wares in great cities as others did, but only take them to the poorer towns, accepting whatever payment people may think they are worth.

Difficulties with self-esteem and depression are common in people with dyslexia (Zausner, 2016) and those with ADHD (Tzelepis et al., 1995). Leonardo may also have seen himself as an outsider because he was born out of wedlock, which carried a social stigma in the Renaissance. His father, Sir Piero, came from an established family in Vinci but never married Leonardo's mother, Catarina, a young woman who lived there. Despite the stress of these conditions, Leonardo went forth into the world and discovered important original information as the result of his observations and analyses.

Leonardo inadvertently shows us that the way we perceive ourselves may be very different from the way we are. Toward the end of his notebooks

(1970b, p. 414), despite his vast accomplishments, Leonardo writes, "Tell me if anything was ever done?" Distressed by concerns that he has not created enough, Leonardo states, "Death before weariness" (1970a, p. 357), and says that no work can tire him. We also see an indomitable resilience in the determination that keeps him going. "Obstacles cannot crush me," he writes (p. 356). "Every obstacle yields to stern resolve," states Leonardo, insisting that, "He who is fixed to a star does not change his mind."

CHAPTER 9

Illness and Transformation in the Creative Trance

Experts are those, who pass through the forest of thorns

Zen Proverb

Art is a wound turned into light

Georges Braque

Just as illness and difficulties punctuate our lives, so do times of triumph and healing. As an experience of renewal and recovery, healing through self-expression and achievement is a creative process and a triumph of the creative trance. When illness brings forth the possibility of new work, a new self, and new aspects of existence, it becomes a transforming illness (Zausner, 2016), an experience of post-traumatic growth, like the deafness of Ludwig van Beethoven (1770–1827) that gave greater power to his music. Healing can occur in organized activities, such as the creative arts therapies, or it may be the experience of an individual, physically and emotionally evolving through creative work. Even when an illness is terminal, creativity may continue in an altered form, generating an internal nonphysical healing that still retains the benefits and profound satisfaction of a creative trance.

The Antiquity and Prevalence of Healing through Creativity

Among the most appreciated and healing aspects of the creative trance are its abilities to address emotional and physical pain and its capacities to express feelings that could not otherwise be articulated (Sandblom, 1997; Zausner, 2016). The connection between creativity and healing is ancient and profound. Dating back millennia in the written record (Horden, 2000; Sonke, 2011), its association most likely existed well before that time. What we now call the creative arts therapies, which comprise healing through the arts and physical movement, are used ritually in nonindustrial

130

cultures today. In these societies, healing is often accompanied by music, dance, and images.

Healing rituals of Native North America, Tibet, and the San Bushmen of Africa (Ricard, 2003; Heeney, 2005; Krippner, 2008) use music and dance to effect positive change for individuals and for the entire society. Ethiopia has an ancient tradition of religious talismanic images, which are venerated as medicinal when viewed (Mercier, 1979, 1997), and in Renaissance Italy (Cardarelli & Fenelli, 2017), images of healing saints were regarded as the source of miraculous cures.

The Creative Trance: Reducing Distress and Facilitating Self-Expression

Creativity can soothe emotional pain and express deep feelings that cannot be communicated in any other way. As the poet William Congreve (1670–1729) observed, "Music hath charms to sooth a savage breast" (2017, Act I, Scene 1). Music can even calm professional musicians. During an interview with the musicologist Elyse Mach (1980, p. 58), the pianist Alicia de Larrocha (1923–2009) revealed, "I have a tendency to be moody at times . . . and the only way out of it is to become completely involved in the music. The music will carry me through." The pianist Andre Watts (b. 1946) also found playing music to be comforting. He explained that "going to the piano and just playing gently and listening to sounds makes everything slowly feel all right" (cited in Gubar, 2020).

The visual artist Georgia O'Keeffe (1887–1986) also soothed herself by playing the piano (Pollitzer, 1988), but found she could express her feelings more fully through painting. Describing an abstract shape on one of her canvases, O'Keeffe (1976) called it "the most definite form for the intangible thing in myself that I can only clarify in paint." The dancer and choreographer Isadora Duncan (1877–1927) expressed her inner self through movement (1997, p. 207), saying, "My Art is just an effort to express the truth of my Being in gesture and movement . . . the most secret impulses of my soul."

The Creative Trance: Diminishing the Experience of Pain

Across domains, the creative trance has effectively lessened the experience of pain. During creativity, the intense focus on work can not only block stimuli from the outside world but may also diminish inner sensations of pain and distress. There appears to be a biological basis for these analgesic qualities. One aspect of creativity's ability for distraction may be explained by gate control theory. This concept sees the brain as a dynamic system, actively selecting, filtering, and modulating its input (Melzack & Wall, 1965; Melzack, 1999). Gate control theory postulates a neurological gate or neuromatrix in the brain, capable of either blocking or receiving stimuli. Possibly during the creative process, positive input inundating the sensory pathways may inhibit sensations of pain, blocking them from reaching the brain and central nervous system.

Some of the positive experiences during creativity may come from its enjoyable state of flow that produces inner satisfaction and a desire to continue the rewarding activity (Csikszentmihalyi, 1990, 1996). In the flow state, where brain waves slow from the beta of everyday interactions down to the alpha waves of relaxation, the body releases a cascade of neurochemicals (Kotler, 2014). Flooding the system with biochemicals that enhance performance while inducing pleasure, it produces dopamine, norepinephrine, anandamide, and serotonin. Other aspects of pain modulation may be the production of beta endorphins during exercise (Heitkamp et al., 1993), and the release of cortisol and endogenous opioids in response to severe physical stress or injury (Melzack, 1999).

The Creative Trance: Lessening Physical Pain across Domains

Distraction from pain, intensity of focus, a release of endogenous chemicals, and a positive response to creative effort appear to combine into a strong palliative response across domains. Dancers perform with both injury pain and performance pain (Anderson & Hanrahan, 2008). In sports (Murphy & White, 1995), football players have finished games despite broken noses, ribs, fingers, and toes; boxers have fought with broken wrists and hands; and distance runners are known to continue their course despite severe pain. The physician and runner Roger Bannister (1929–2018) described his creative trance state as having "no pain only a great unity of movement and aim" (2018, p. 171). The centenarian champion runner Ida Olivia Keeling (1915-2021) had arthritis and sometimes walked with a cane, but always ran without one (Remnick & Berenstein, 2016).

Visual artists also use the creative trance as an analgesic (Zausner, 2016). After a severe traffic accident at age eighteen left Frida Kahlo (1907–1954) in bed with pain from multiple injuries, she turned to art. Henri de Toulouse-Lautrec (1864–1901), who was born with pycnodysostosis, an inherited disease that causes brittle bones, multiple fractures, and severe sinus problems, turned to art in childhood to distract himself from the pain. The folk artist Maud Lewis (1903–1970), who had pain from severe juvenile arthritis that continued throughout her life, said (cited in Woolaver, 1995, p. 29), "As long as I've got a brush in front of me, I'm all right."

The Northern Sung dynasty painter Li Kung-lin (1040–1106), known also as Li Lung-mien, insisted on making art, even when he was old, bedridden, and in pain (Binyon, 1969). No longer able to manage a brush, Li Kung-lin used his severely arthritic hands to make lines on the bedsheets. An onlooker might only see creases in the linens, but in Li Kung-lin's creative trance they were paintings as beautiful as those he once made with brush and ink.

Expressive Arts Therapies and the Healing Creative Trance

With its analgesic qualities and deep expressive capacities, the creative trance is central to healing modalities across cultures and domains. In contemporary society, healing through art is the focus of the expressive arts therapies (Serlin, 2007; Samaritter, 2018); they include: art therapy, dance therapy, music therapy, writing therapy, poetry therapy, drama therapy, and in sports there is equine-assisted therapy. Using creativity to release, express, and examine unconscious feelings and emotional pain, the expressive arts therapies are now mainstream healing modalities. Self-disclosure through creativity is therapeutic, can benefit the immune system, and reduce feelings of isolation (Gabora, 2017).

The work created becomes a tool for self-knowledge, bringing up material from the unconscious mind and concretizing it into a tangible item or activity. Here, the creative trance and its products, although initially generated by a creative individual, are shared with a professional, who assists with insights and guidance. In accessing the unconscious mind nonverbally, expressive arts therapies may uncover material not readily available in talk therapy, which can be useful in populations with limited verbal communication.

Dance Therapy and the Healing Embodied Mutual Creative Trance

Expressive arts therapies allow traumatized individuals to experience emotional release through dance and movement, an embodied type of creative arts therapy which has become an internationally accepted method of healing (Serlin, 2010; Levine & Land, 2016). The psychologist Ilene

Serlin (b. 1948), who is also a dancer and dance therapist, has used dance as an embodied expressive arts therapy in Israel, Turkey, Jordan, and China. In June of 2019, the International Existential Humanistic Institute at Peking University Hospital in Beijing China invited Serlin (2022) to give a training demonstration at their psychiatric center for eating disorders. There were approximately forty psychiatrists and other medical doctors in the room, who had come to learn about incorporating embodied creative arts therapy into their practices.

The patient, M, who volunteered for the session and spoke English, was a very thin young woman age twenty-two, with a history of multiple hospital admissions due to anorexia and bulimia. This time, after fainting at home, M was brought to the hospital's ICU. Her teeth were severely damaged from vomiting and she had almost died. M's mother was weeping in despair in the next room. Serlin was told that M liked to dance, and M chose a Chinese folk dance for the demonstration. She agreed to dance with Serlin, and as they danced opposite each other, M showed Serlin the dance steps. At first M moved stiffly, but then she became more rhythmic and fluid. Reaching out her hands to take Serlin's hands, M indicated nonverbally the directions in which they should move.

Birth of a New Self in the Healing Embodied Creative Trance

When the well-known Chinese peacock dance came on the tape, M lifted and fluttered her arms, revealing lyrical and poetic aspects of herself. Serlin said she shadowed M's movements, joining only when invited. Then came a rocking motion with bent arms that M called *baby*. It became apparent that they were taking care of a sleeping baby that they gently caressed and placed on the ground. Several minutes went by. Then M looked at Serlin, saying, "I want to change, I want to change my life" (2019). Serlin answered, "You can," and M said, "I can," and Serlin responded, "You will." As they both continued to stroke the baby, M said, "I want to make my family happy," and Serlin replied, "You can."

Then M asked to hear a lullaby and Serlin had a well-known Chinese lullaby on her tape. While the music played, Serlin saw that many of the doctors in the room had tears flowing down their faces. The hushed atmosphere felt sacred. Now, as they were nearing the end of the session, Serlin softly asked M if she would like to take her baby. As they gently lifted the baby into M's arms, she said to Serlin, "I'm hungry. I want to eat." Then they told each other they would always remember this time. Serlin, who had tears in her eyes, recognized they were her wishes for M's continued well-being and for the gratitude and privilege of working as a healer.

The Transforming Illness and the Creative Trance

Whatever affects our body has the capacity to alter our creative trance. While the expressive arts therapies have formalized techniques for healing through creativity, artists have a history of healing themselves with their work. As the writer and physician Rachel Naomi Remen (cited in Corley, 2010, p. 543) says, "At the deepest level, the creative process and the healing process arise from a single source. When you are an artist, you are a healer." While it may seem paradoxical, sometimes the most severe physical illnesses can change creativity for the better. The experience can be a type of "transformation through suffering" (Taylor, 2012, p. 30). When this happens, a time of poor health becomes what I call a *transforming illness* (Zausner, 2016) because it alters a creative person's life and work.

Ethnic Origins, Healing, and the Creative Trance

There are potentially as many instances of transforming illnesses as there are people in poor health, but this section will focus on artists who turned to their ethnic heritage as a source of strength and inspiration in their creative trance. They combined an established tradition with their own originality, and in doing so had an experience of healing. The creative trance is a playground for the unconscious mind and using an ethnic heritage as structure acts as a scaffolding for the unconscious to bring forth the surprising and the new. This experience can be psychologically strengthening and healing for a creative person because working in an ethnic heritage brings with it an ancient and inherent sense of approval. With this ground of acceptance, the artist becomes a conduit from a respected past to a creative present.

Itchiku Kubota: Reinventing a Tradition of Japanese Textiles and Kimonos

The textile artist and kimono designer Itchiku Kubota (1917–2003) turned to his ethnic heritage twice for inspiration and recovery. At age nineteen, when Kubota (1984) was working for a company engaged in the classic yūzen style of dyeing kimonos, he collapsed from overwork and exhaustion. Yet this physical crisis generated a turning point in his life. Afterward, Kubota opened his own kimono studio and began to study the ancient, almost forgotten tsuijigahana style of fabric dyeing. Kubota eventually combined the two styles and at age sixty had a first exhibition and a second one scheduled for the following year.

On the day of his second exhibition, he became seriously ill with acute hepatitis. Yet, "this was the time of deepest import in my life as an artist," insists Kubota (1984, p. 129). "For the next two months, I struggled against death," he said. "While in the hospital I thought over all I had done and decided to turn to developing my own style." After his illness Kubota gained great success by reinterpreting classical Japanese techniques and designs in contemporary fabrics and colors, while also bringing in images of nature and influences from French Impressionism.

Richard Yarde: African and African American Healing

In 1991, the visual artist Richard Yarde (1939–2011) had kidney failure in response to his high blood pressure medication. The reaction also produced stroke-like symptoms that impaired his mobility, slurred his speech, and left him without feeling in both hands (Worcester Art Museum, 2003a, 2003b; Yarde, 2006; UMass Amherst, 2011; Zausner, 2016). Although Yarde said his doctors expected him to die, he was determined to live and make art. After a year of intensive rehabilitation, he was able to speak correctly, feel his hands, and move again. Even though Yarde had to sleep connected to a dialysis machine until his kidney transplant in 1998, he returned to work as a professor of art at the University of Massachusetts and to painting.

In coming back to art, Yarde said he wanted to heal himself further through creativity. Yarde had previously used the dance and music of his African American heritage as inspiration, but now he went back to its beginnings. He focused on the enslaved origins of African Americans in the United States and their fight to preserve their African culture. It is possible that Yarde further identified with the early African American struggle for cultural preservation because of his personal battle for self-preservation.

The work he created is a series of large watercolors based on *Ringshout*, a circle dance that African Americans brought with them from Africa. It was used for healing, community solidarity, and spiritual transformation. Prohibited from having instruments, the slaves created rhythms for the ritual by clapping their hands and stomping their feet. Symbolizing the dancers' feet by modern shoes as they moved around the circle, Yarde also included X-rays, acupuncture, DNA patterns, and ultrasounds into his images, bringing a historical healing ceremony into the medical present. The composition of the *Ringshout* paintings is also healing. As a circular dance, set within a square canvas, it creates a mandala, which Jung (1972) cites as an archetypal symbol of wholeness.

Ernie Pepion: Native American Traditions and Advocacy for the Disabled

"I am an artist, Blackfeet Indian, and am physically disabled," stated Ernie Eewokso Pepion (1943–2005) (1993, n.p.), who used his work to expose prejudice against the disabled and people of color. "Through painting I show my experience of these degradations," said Pepion (1993, n.p.). He even expressed this through his signature, where the last three letters of his name *Pepion* combine to form an image of a wheelchair.

Before the accident and its aftermath that became his transforming illness (Zausner, 2016), Pepion worked on his family's ranch in Montana and was a rider in rodeos. Then in 1971, four years after returning home as a decorated war hero, Pepion was in the passenger seat of a car that crashed and broke his spine, leaving him quadriplegic (Kumpf, 1993). Initially treated in a Montana hospital, he was transferred to a California Veterans Administration Hospital that specialized in spinal injuries. While he was there, Pepion learned to paint from a man who was in an iron lung because of polio. The man could only leave the iron lung for one hour per day, and he spent that hour painting. Pepion wanted to paint too, but his right hand was weak. In response, the hospital made him a hand/forearm brace to support the hand and enable him to hold a brush.

After returning home, Pepion enrolled in Montana State University as an art major, graduating with honors for his bachelor's and master's degree. While he was there, the engineering department created a motorized wheelchair that would help him when he worked on large canvases. Until his death from illness in 2005, Pepion created paintings that fused his dreams with reality (Lippard, 1993), exteriorizing his longings, which were the motivating factors of his creative trance. In this altered state Pepion no longer felt pejoritized and was able to express himself more fully. He said (1993, n.p.), "Painting allows me to be a person beyond the limits of racial prejudice and disability. Art enables me to address feelings that are difficult for me to write or even talk about."

In one painting, Pepion is doing a Native American dance, half standing out of his wheelchair, which he could not do in waking life, yet acknowledging his physical limitations by holding the chair's arm for support. In another painting, wanting to ride again but physically unable, Pepion shows himself galloping on a horse with his wheelchair blended into its sides, so that he, the horse, and the wheelchair have become one. This image, which may seem paradoxical to the conscious mind, is an accepted reality in the altered state of a creative trance. While the oneness of the wheelchair, the horse, and the rider is not possible in the physics of waking consciousness, through their painted union, Pepion reveals the emotional truth of a profound inner experience.

When the Creative Trance during Illness Reveals a Destiny in Art

There are instances when the stimulus for a creative trance is received so strongly that the altered state it generates brings a profound recognition of the person's destined path in life. For the visual artists Henri Matisse and Albert Pinkham Ryder, this happened during a time of illness.

Henri Matisse (1869–1954) had five transforming illnesses (Zausner, 2016), but it was the first one that changed his career path from law to art. Matisse, who had no interest in law, entered the profession as the result of family pressure. When he was a young lawyer the chronic gastrointestinal problems he had since childhood flared up and became acute, necessitating a stay in the hospital (Flam, 1986; Sandblom, 1997). In the next bed, there was a man doing chromos, which are an early type of painting-by-numbers. Matisse asked his mother to buy him one, and when she brought him two small chromos with a paint set, he immediately entered an altered state. "The moment I had this box of colors in my hands," said Matisse (cited in Flam, 1986, pp. 27–28), "I had the feeling that my life was there." Before this time, nothing interested him, but from that event onward, he focused only on art.

Albert Pinkham Ryder (1847–1917) was a quiet child who enjoyed making art since he was age four (Brown, 1989; Homer & Goodrich, 1989). While still in grade school, Ryder developed a severe reaction to a vaccination that inflamed his eyes. It was most likely a smallpox vaccination because he grew up in the seaport town of New Bedford, Massachusetts, which had a policy of enforcing smallpox vaccinations to control its repeated outbreaks (Ellis, 1892; Tucker, 2001). Although the boy was sick with weakened sight, his compassionate father bought him art supplies. In response, Ryder had a creative trance foreseeing his destiny.

"When my father placed a box of colors and brushes in my hands and I stood before my easel with its square of stretched canvas," said Ryder. "I realized that I had in my possession the wherewith to create a masterpiece that would live throughout the coming ages."

Beethoven and Hearing Loss

Sensory impairments, such as hearing loss can also become a transforming illness. Currently 466 million people worldwide, or more than 5 percent of our population, have a disabling hearing impairment (WHO, 2020). Perhaps the most famous creative person with profound hearing loss is the composer and pianist Ludwig van Beethoven (1770–1827).

Beethoven's hearing problems, which started in his left ear and then included his right, appeared to consist of three types: nerve deafness (Huxtable, 2001; Saccenti et al., 2011), tinnitus, and hyperacusis (Huxtable, 2001). In his early years Beethoven had excellent hearing and was a musical prodigy who gave a concert at age seven and published a musical composition at age twelve. Yet by age twenty-seven he began to have diminished sound discrimination and an inability to hear sounds of a high pitch, which are symptoms of nerve deafness.

By 1801 Beethoven had developed hyperacusis, an uncomfortable hyper-sensitivity to upper-and lower-threshold sounds. With this condition, both squeaking and coughing may be painful to hear. At that time and onward, Beethoven (2008, n.p.) also had tinnitus, saying "my ears are buzzing and ringing perpetually, day and night."

Beethoven: Deafness as a Transforming Illness

The deafness that isolated Beethoven became a transforming illness; it influenced his music and gave him more time to compose. With diminished hearing Beethoven was no longer able to be a concert pianist or conduct orchestras. He also withdrew from social life because he could not hear. At first Beethoven tried to hide his deafness from others, but as his hearing loss increased and could not be hidden, he used conversation books, a type of notebook, to communicate by writing.

With relentlessly encroaching deafness, Beethoven self-isolated, devoting more of his solitary time to music. In a creative trance, his hearing loss was not as upsetting as it was in social circumstances. As he wrote in a letter (2008), "My affliction is less distressing when playing and composing, and most so in intercourse with others." With this intensity of work in his lifetime of fifty-six years, Beethoven created nine symphonies, five piano concertos, one opera, thirty-two piano sonatas, one violin concerto, and seventeen string quartets (Kubba & Young, 1996).

The influence of deafness is apparent in his music, where compositions are grouped into three main periods (Kubba & Young, 1996). The music of the first period, which extends to 1800 during the early symptoms of his hearing problems, shows the influence of Haydn, Mozart, and other previous composers. In the middle period, 1800–1815, Beethoven's deafness increased. Unable to actively hear the work of other composers, his music becomes more his own with the Moonlight Sonata and four symphonies. During the last period, 1816–1827, when Beethoven was almost completely deaf, and had severe emotional and physical problems, such as debilitating gastrointestinal illnesses, he wrote the Missa Solemnis, six string quartets, piano sonatas, and his powerful Ninth Symphony (Huxtable, 2000).

The intensity of Beethoven's physical and emotional pain was transmogrified into his passion for music and this passion communicated itself to others. The composer Wilhelm Richard Wagner (1813–1883) regarded the late works as Beethoven's ultimate achievement, saying, "Beethoven's Ninth Symphony became the mystical goal of all my strange thoughts and desires about music" (Wagner, 2004a, K. L. 662). Wagner, who translated the Ninth Symphony into a piano concerto, revealed (K. L. 667–668) that it seemed "to form the spiritual keynote of my own life."

Beethoven, Hearing Loss, and the Importance of the Creative Trance

The creative trance is important for everyone. Yet when a person's world is narrowed through illness, pain, and sensory deprivation, as it was for Beethoven, then the creative trance may assume an even greater and sometimes lifesaving role. "Live only for your art, for you are so limited by your senses," he said (cited in Huxtable, 2001, p. 11). In his letters (Beethoven, 2008, K., n.p.) we see anguish, devotion to his work, and multiple thoughts of suicide that are only abated through creativity. "How often have I cursed my existence!" Beethoven exclaims. But then he thanks "Art for not having ended my life by suicide." Beethoven insists that even though he was on "the verge of desperation . . . Art! Art alone, deterred me. Ah! how could I possibly quit the world before bringing forth all that I felt it was my vocation to produce?"

Beethoven's musical creative trance had become a lifeline, but by 1812 his hearing had significantly diminished. To amplify sound so that he could continue composing, Beethoven turned to the technology of his day. He had Johann Nepomuk Mälzel (1772–1838), inventor of the metronome, make four ear trumpets for him, two with head bands to free his hands for playing music (Huxtable, 2001). In 1817, he requested a piano with increased volume from the piano maker Andreas (Saccenti et al., 2011). Beethoven also ordered a resonance plate from the pianoforte company of Conrad Graf (Ealy, 1994). A resonance plate is a type of sound conductor that can be placed on top of a piano. Ealy (1994) believes that Beethoven put the bowl end of his largest ear trumpet on the resonance plate to capture the piano sounds while he was composing.

Several people attested to Beethoven's use of a resonance plate, but there was one uncorroborated report by Rattel (Ealy, 1994; Kubba & Young, 1996) that said Beethoven used a wooden drumstick held in his teeth to hear the music he played. The round ball at the end of the stick possibly touched the piano sending sound vibrations to his teeth and then on to the bones of the middle ear for hearing, bypassing the outer ears. Even in his later years, Beethoven was never completely deaf; he had a very small amount of hearing in his left ear. This residual hearing was like a minuscule opening in a wall of deafness, but through this opening he composed his major late works. It became a minute hole in what was previously thought to be an impervious wall, yet looking through it, one can see the whole world.

Hearing Loss and the Creative Trance in Visual Artists

While hearing loss is central to a creative person in music, it can also affect the lives and work of visual artists. Throughout the centuries, there have been visual artists with hearing loss progressing to partial or complete deafness (Sonnenstrahl, 2003). Sometimes, as with the painter Joshua Reynolds (1723–1792), who used his hearing difficulty as a way of avoiding people he disliked, it did not make a significant impact on an already established career. Yet with other painters, such as Charlotte Buell Coman and Francisco Goya, hearing loss transformed their creative trance and their lives.

The landscape painter Charlotte Buell Coman (1833–1924) showed an early ability for visual art, but it was not until she was age forty and losing her hearing that that she turned to painting as a profession (Sonnenstrahl, 2002). Coman, who then studied art in Europe for ten years, was influenced by the quiet nostalgic images of the French Barbizon painters. While her misty blue-green landscapes, which convey a mood of *quietism*, may reflect the artist's increasingly quiet world (Zausner, 2016), their visual calmness may also have been therapeutic for Coman and for viewers. As Coman's creative trance seems to incorporate calmness, Francisco Goya's creative trance appears to be powered by rage.

Francisco Goya (Francisco de Goya y Lucientes, 1746–1828) suffered an acute debilitating illness in 1792 (Descargues, 1979; de Salas, 1981). He had been in failing health with blackouts and hallucinations, but now Goya became sick for months with partial paralysis, vision problems, deafness, a loss of balance, and confusion. Eventually his symptoms abated except for a profound deafness that left him, at age forty-six, with a constant roaring and buzzing in his ears. Before his illness, Goya painted light, colorful rococo paintings on commission, but afterward he painted increasingly for himself. His production increased and his work became darker, more structured, political, and psychological. As his work changed, it strengthened, and Goya became a romantic painter, a precursor to modern art.

Using a Creative Trance to Heal the World: Greta Thunberg

There are times when a person will intentionally use the creative trance to rectify social and environmental problems. Intuitively realizing the healing power of creative work, she hopes to inspire others toward action. The aim is to generate an influential audience creative trance that will produce a large-scale response. Then the creativity that begins as a personal concept will expand to improve conditions for an entire society. There is enormous creativity in having a sense of purpose; it marshals both mental and physical resources in multiple and often original ways to achieve a goal.

A sense of purpose transformed Greta Tintin Eleonora Ernman Thunberg (b. 2003) from an isolated schoolgirl into a hero for climate change (Sengupta, 2019; Thunberg, 2019a, 2019b). "I'm happier now," said Thunberg. "I have meaning. I have something I have to do" (cited in Sengupta, 2019, n.p.). Having a cause greater than herself brought Thunberg out of her small personal world and into the larger world that we share, the world that she is trying to heal. She did this by turning her greatest weakness into her greatest strength. Evolving from someone with a crippling anxiety about speaking at all, Thunberg now gives speeches worldwide on climate change.

Thunberg (2019a, 2019b, n.p.) has Asperger's syndrome, which under "the right circumstances" she believes can be like a "superpower." Yet in school it caused her to be isolated and bullied to the extent that, at age eleven, she went into a severe depression, stopped attending classes, stopped eating, and ceased to grow. Thunberg also developed selective mutism, an anxiety disorder where speech is extremely limited. She spoke only to her family and to one teacher at school. Otherwise, she was silent. Yet the anxiety that Thunberg felt about global warming, the melting ice caps, the fires, and the injured wildlife, which had been growing inside her since she was age eight, eventually became greater than the anxiety that maintained her silence.

Climate change has compelled her to talk. The words she had suppressed came out on social media, creating a following with students around the world who joined her in school strikes for reduced carbon emissions. Words are her greatest strength, aiming for a creative trance of intense audience persuasion in speeches to the United Nations, the World Economic Forum, the Austrian Summit, and elsewhere. In 2019 Thunberg was nominated for a Nobel Peace Prize and Time magazine chose her as Person of the Year.

The Final Illness and the Creative Trance: Jacqueline du Pré

The creative trance is an interior state that is outwardly expressed in works of art. Even when illness prevents a person from physically concretizing their creativity, the work and its creative trance lives on in their consciousness. As a result, the desire for self-expression can be so strong that it may compel a person to completely alter their usual mode of working in order to remain creative (Zausner, 2016). This is most clearly expressed in the final illness, where creative people will struggle against great and increasing difficulties to remain creative for as long as they can.

Like the brief flashing arc of a shooting star, the career of cellist Jacqueline du Pré (1945–1987) started with brilliance and prizes but continued only to age twenty-eight, ended by multiple sclerosis (Curtin, 2015). Yet du Pré carried the music inside her and even with the many physical infirmities of multiple sclerosis, she struggled to continue performing. Despite the growing inability to control her hands and the increasing numbness in her fingers to the point where she could no longer sense the strings of her cello or feel the weight of her bow, du Pré continued to play by visually perceiving her hand positions and listening to the music (Tierradentro-García et al., 2018). Finally, no longer able to perform, du

Pré expressed her creativity through teaching others when her condition allowed this.

Creativity can be so important to individuals that they, like du Pré, will change domains because of illness or other incapacity, to remain creatively productive. Changing domains to continue the experience of a creative trance is a well-known occurrence in the visual arts, where painting or traveling for photojournalism can require an ongoing stamina that may not be available in poor health or older age (Zausner, 2016). When Parkinson's prevented the photojournalist Margaret Bourke-White (1904–1971) from traveling for assignments, she focused on writing. The visual artist Cecilia Beaux (1855–1942) wrote an autobiography, *Background with Figures*, after breaking her hip in a fall that stopped her from painting. The visual artist and naturalist Albrecht Dürer (1471–1528) turned increasingly to writing in the last years of his life when he was sick with malaria.

The Final Illness and the Creative Trance: John Mallord William Turner

Even with a limited capacity for physical movement, the creative trance can be profoundly fulfilling. It can create beautiful works of art in the artist's imagination that transcend the constraints and ailments of the physical world. This, apparently, was the experience of the painter John Mallord William Turner (1775–1851).

In the last months of his life, when his heart was failing, Turner secretly left his home in London for his Chelsea cottage near the River Thames (Finberg, 1967; Hamilton, 1997). On the roof of the cottage there was a balcony with a view of both the sunrise and sunset on the boats and water that were the subjects of his art. Too weak to do extensive painting, Turner instead became an observer. This contemplative absorption of stimuli is the receptive side of a creative trance (Zausner, 2016). Turner's view was beautiful, and beauty is information. It is possible that Turner was processing this information as if it were to be translated onto a canvas, although he was increasingly unable to paint. Artists tend to do this even though they may not be painting at that moment or might, like Turner, not be able to paint again. Some masterpieces are created only to be seen in the mind.

CHAPTER 10

Different Abilities and the Creative Trance

The impediment to action advances the action. What stands in the way becomes the way

Marcus Aurelius

The key to your personal transformation is the thorn in your side

Rudolph Ballentine

Challenges can become opportunities to excel, and different abilities enlarge the terrain of the creative trance. While not every condition can be "cured," healing is always available through self-transformation. Individuals in this chapter have a double creative trance. In addition to the altered state in performing sports, Paralympic competitions, dance, wheelchair dance, music, science, and visual art, sometimes without limbs, vision, or hearing, they share a specific kind of creative trance that cuts across domains. They share a triumph of achievement gained through accomplishing something that was at one time thought to be impossible – perhaps even by them.

Overcoming the Impossible: Different Abilities and the Creative Trance

You might ask why include a discussion about disabilities and the creative trance. Aren't the Paralympic participants athletes, aren't the wheelchair performers dancers, aren't the blind musicians musicians, and aren't the differently abled painters visual artists – and shouldn't they be in the chapters of this book specific to their domains? Of course, they are athletes, dancers, musicians, and visual artists and share in the creative trance of their domains. Yet the extra effort needed to confront impediments makes their creative determination so powerful that it transforms their lives and alters the neural landscapes of their brains.

Concerted effort and focused aim made their impossible possible and that is the nature of their creative trance. In achieving goals, they widen the possibilities for everyone by demonstrating the extended capacities of human beings. We humans, like all other animals, are a species with varied abilities. Yet until recently, this had not been officially acknowledged. Although blindness and musical ability have a long history (Rowden, 2012), now the Paralympics, visual art by the blind, and wheelchair dancing are part of modern culture. In a creative trance, the differently abled can focus away from impediments and onto their inner wholeness and capacity to excel.

A cure eliminates a physical illness or condition, but healing strengthens us from within even without a physical cure. Often in healing, what was previously considered to be an impediment becomes the foundation for higher achievement. This happens when difficulties inspire strength, motivation, and more psychologically integrated functioning. What we must overcome becomes an opportunity to succeed.

Dance Trance for the Differently Abled

Legs are no longer necessary for dancing. David Vincent Toole (1964–2020), possibly the world's best-known disabled dancer, had his legs amputated at the age of eighteen months because of sacral agenesis (Hadoke, 2020; Marano, 2020). This inherited condition affects fetal development, causing malformation of the lower spine and the legs. Without needing legs, Toole was a highly expressive dancer and actor, lifting his body easily and gracefully with strong arms and enormous hands that were also capable of very delicate movements. These abilities were evident in his performance at the opening of the 2012 London Paralympic Games. After starting to dance on stage, Toole was lifted twenty-two meters high, far above the stadium and its audience. In this aerial routine he fluidly moved his arms and hands, simulating wings and enhancing the illusion of flight.

Born in Leeds, Toole worked in the postal service as a young man, until he decided to take a weeklong dance workshop for people of all abilities. When he initially told his mother of his plan, she responded, "Can I just remind you that you don't have any legs" (cited in Hadoke, 2020). Yet, the dance trance can be extremely compelling, and after the workshop, dance and then also acting became the focus of his life. Toole left his postal position and moved to London. There he went to the Trinity Laban Conservatoire of Music and Dance, and worked at the Candoco Dance

Company, which integrates abled and disabled dancers. Toole performed in the theater, Shakespeare plays, films, and television, and was at the Stopgap Dance Company, which includes the disabled and the abled, when he was awarded an OBE (Officer of the Order of the British Empire) (ArtsProfessional, 2020).

Toole's honor came for his contributions to dance and to people with disabilities. Lucy Bennett, the Artistic Director of Stopgap Dance Company, applauded Toole's award, calling him a role model for disabled and nondisabled dancers. She said (cited in Marano, 2020), "We cannot underestimate the huge difference he has made to disabled dancers who have followed in his handprints instead of the steps of nondisabled dancers. The world is beginning to become more inclusive thanks to Dave."

Dance Trance and the Wheelchair

David Toole, more widely known for his hand dancing, also danced using a wheelchair. The wheelchair, in either its manual or powered version, has become a dance vehicle for professional and recreational dancers, for those in dance therapy, and for para dance athletes at the Paralympics (2020b). Wheelchair dance, which began in 1968 and became a sport of the International Paralympic Committee in 1998, has four main formats (Inal, 2014). There is combi-dance, where a wheelchair dancer and an able-bodied dancer perform together; duo-dance, where both dancers use wheelchairs; group dance, where multiple wheelchair users and able-bodied dancers dance together; and single dance, which is a solo performance by a dancer in a wheelchair.

In addition to the documented physical, emotional, and social benefits of dance (Earhart, 2009; Serlin, 2010; Dewhurst et al., 2014), there can be an intense attachment to the experience of a dance creative trance. The intensity of the dance trance, which has been used cross-culturally in ecstatic religious rituals, may bring a sense of transcendence, empowerment, and joy into secular life. When the classically trained ballet dancer Mehmet Sefa Ozturk became paraplegic after a motorcycle accident, he changed to para dance sport at the Paralympics (2020a) and declared, "I never gave up dancing." The world champion wheelchair dancer Piotr Iwanicki (b. 1984) reveals his creative trance, saying, "When I'm on the dance floor, nothing matters at all. Dancing is all my life. It's my passion" (cited in Li, 2017). Iwanicki, who is also a civil engineer, was born with spina bifida, and has been using a wheelchair all his life. He teaches dance, saying, "It doesn't matter if you are using crutches, wheelchair, power chair, you can always dance."

International Physically Integrated Dance and Theater Companies

Dance, theater, and their compelling creative trances are now increasingly available to disabled people. Part of a growing movement in contemporary culture, they are also known as physically integrated, inclusive, or differently abled dance and theater. A leading organization promoting disabled artists is Europe Beyond Access, co-funded by the European Commission's Creative Europe program (British Council, 2020). The seven trans-European core partners of Europe Beyond Access are the British Council, which operates this project in the United Kingdom and in Poland, the Holland Dance Festival in the Netherlands, Per.Art in Serbia, Kampnagel in Germany, Onassis Stegi in Greece, Oriente Occidente in Italy, and Skånes Dansteater in Sweden. In the United States, there is the AXIS Dance Company of Oakland, California (2020) and Infinite Flow in Los Angeles (Hamamoto, 2020), among others.

Physically integrated dance and theater companies bring together people of all abilities, including those using wheelchairs, able-bodied individuals, and performers with protheses, who have the option of whether to wear them or not. Including everyone can generate feelings of unconditional acceptance, that may possibly have aspects in common with feelings of unconditional love. Feelings of acceptance are important for everyone, especially for those individuals who may have previously been marginalized by prejudice. As motivating and energizing for a creative trance, the exuberant acceptance of self and group found in inclusive dance and theater companies is expanding the boundaries of the creative process. Dance can also increase mobility and improve quality of life for individuals with Parkinson's, as seen in Dance for PD (2020), which offers dance classes for people with Parkinson's.

The Immobile Dance Trance: Marissa Hamamoto

The wheelchair dancer Piotr Iwanicki has combi-dance partnered with the able-bodied professional ballroom dancer Marissa Hamamoto (b. 1982). Their duet *Gravity* can be seen online at Infinite Flow, a ballroom dance company that Hamamoto (2020) founded in Los Angeles based on the principles of diversity and inclusion: for people of all backgrounds and abilities. In 2006 Hamamoto suffered a spinal cord infarction, which is a form of stroke in the spine, that paralyzed her from the neck down. Yet as one of the inspirations for her dance company, it became a transforming illness. When the doctors told Hamamoto she would never walk again, she insisted, "Even if I cannot walk again, I will find a way to dance, even if it were from a wheelchair" (cited in Li, 2017).

While paralyzed in the hospital, Hamamoto received physical and occupational therapy but also used visualization, an aspect of the creative trance, to see herself as a fully functioning dancer. She continually imagined herself dancing, repeating complex ballet sequences she had learned, and activating her brain to the sensation of movement (Li, 2017). Within a month, she was walking again. Mizuguchi and associates (2012) find that visualization is beneficial in sports performance and in rehabilitation from physical problems. They suggest a possible reason for this benefit is that vivid imagery and complex movements during visualization may increase excitability in the corticospinal pathway. This tract of nerve fibers that descends from the cortex into the spine controls voluntary movements from the neck down to the feet (Van Wittenberghe & Peterson, 2020).

There also appears to be a type of "functional equivalence" between visualized and physically activated movements (Kilteni et al., 2018). Visualized movements have been able to increase biological markers, such as heart rate, in proportion to the intensity of the visualized efforts, as do physically initiated movements. In addition, visualization appears to activate a group of brain networks, including the frontal motor areas, cerebellar regions, and parietal areas that are partially congruent with brain networks active during physical actions.

Wheelchair Dancing for Children: A Dance Trance of Transformation

Wheelchair dancing can be a very positive and strengthening experience for children and adolescents with physical disabilities (Goodwin et al., 2004; de Villiers et al., 2013). In their study of a weekly wheelchair dance class in Canada for five children (four girls and one boy), ages six to fourteen, Goodwin, Krohn, and Kuhnle (2004) found the children gained both physical and psychological benefits. All the young dancers had myelomeningocele spina bifida. Three of them had lesions at the lumbar level and two had thoracic-level lesions. All the participants used a wheelchair full time. The study indicated that while the children experienced muscle strengthening, greater flexibility, improved coordination, and better balance, they also gained important psychological benefits.

In addition to the socialization and cooperation through teamwork necessary for pair and group dance combinations, the young dancers showed improved self-confidence and greater self-esteem from having a new path of self-expression. In a creative trance, wheelchairs are implements of dance, an extension of the body, like ice skates for skaters. No longer a symbol of disability, the wheelchair becomes an outlet for emotional and physical self-expression, a vehicle for creative imagination and personal transformation. Wheelchair dancing can reconstruct the concept of an ideal body through movements and their meaning (Goodwin et al., 2004). The young dancers did twirls and pirouettes in their wheelchairs. One dancer said she felt graceful and beautiful, and another said she felt like a star. Jody, age six, revealed, "I feel free like a bird when I dance" (cited in Goodwin et al., 2004, p. 240). In her creative trance she was flying.

The young dancers gave public performances throughout the year to positive audience responses. In their creative trance, "the children expressed thoughts of being one with their wheelchairs, one with the dance, one with each other, and one with the audience" (cited in Goodwin et al., 2004, p. 244). In response, they generated a strong audience creative trance. Some people in the audience were moved to tears, and others said it changed the way they perceived people in wheelchairs. One person wrote (cited in Goodwin et al., 2004, p. 244), "Suddenly I could see these children in a new and beautiful way. My eyes were opened to my own prejudice! Thanks for helping provide a life changing experience."

Paralympic Athletes: A Sports Trance Extending to Achievement and Compassion

The self-expression, accomplishment, and sense of personal power arising during a sports creative trance can impact and empower an athlete's life off court. This is especially true for differently abled athletes, who are in a constant battle with what was previously thought to be impossible. Using the drive, focus, goal-setting behavior, and experiences of self-efficacy that power their sports trance, some of the athletes transform what appear to be insurmountable odds into continued life achievement. It may also be the motivated aspect of their personality and a strong sense of self that brought them into competitive sports. A number of these athletes extend their achievement beyond sports, into activities of compassion. Possibly arising from an empathic identification with other disabled individuals, compassion can be a life-shaping trajectory.

Paralympic Swimmers: Zorn-Hudson and Suzuki

Swimmer Trischa Zorn-Hudson (b. 1964), who won fifty-five medals in seven Paralympic Games, making her the most decorated athlete in its history, taught disabled inner-city school children (Mcleod, 1995; Gawley & Palmer, 2013). She said (cited in Mcleod, 1995, n.p.), "I thought with what I have overcome with my disability that if I could just reach these children in the inner city . . . that I could be a good role model for them." Zorn-Hudson, who was born legally blind due to aniridia, a genetic condition in which the irises of the eyes do not form, focused on sports since childhood. Perseverance, competition, and the enjoyment of challenge shape her sports creative trance. "I really enjoy competing, and swimming seemed to offer that more than anything else I knew," says Zorn-Hudson. She also likes "doing things that are a challenge . . . my best *and* my worse quality is my stubbornness. I'll do something until I get it right" (cited in Ludovise, 1986, n.p.). Zorn-Hudson later went back to school for a law degree and now works as a pro bono lawyer, using the focused qualities of her sports career to help those in need who cannot afford to pay legal fees.

Paralympic swimmer and multiple medal winner Takayuki Suzuki (b. 1987) says, "Ideally, when my swimming career ends, I'd like to work for an organization relating to disability in sport . . . I would like to pass on what I have learned and share my experiences" (cited in Sheridan, 2018, n.p.). Suzuki, who was born with congenital limb deficiency, does not have a right leg, his left leg ends at mid-thigh, and his right arm goes only to his elbow (Sheridan, 2018; Suzuki, 2020). Yet even as a child, Suzuki was drawn to sports. He played football wearing shoes on his hands and enjoyed baseball. As an adult, Suzuki wants to break records, and in his creative trance, he concentrates on a podium finish at the Paralympic Games. Suzuki's creativity also extends to music (Sheridan, 2018; Barber, 2020). In school, he played the French horn and now plays the ichigo-ichie, a Japanese string instrument like a guitar. Suzuki's right arm ends at his elbow, so he invented an extension device that holds the pick allowing him to play. In 2013 Suzuki moved from Japan to the United Kingdom and now lives in Newcastle, where he is studying for a master's degree in International Sports Management from Northumbria University, and plans to continue for his PhD.

Paralympic Wheelchair Rugby Athlete: Bob Lujano

As the medal-winning quadriplegic athlete Bob Lujano (b. 1970) says, "Since I lost my limbs, society has tried to define me. I've gone from crippled to handicapped, to physically challenged, and now to disabled. As far as I'm concerned, I've always just been Bob" (Lujano & Schiro, 2014, n.p.). A Paralympic wheelchair rugby player, Lujano contracted meningococcemia at age nine, a type of meningitis that necessitated the amputation of his arms beneath the elbow and his legs below the knee. In the hospital bed after his amputations, Lujano had a profound near death experience that remains a vivid memory. "I'm talking to Jesus. I'm telling him to leave me here because I have things to do," said Lujano (Lujano & Schiro, 2014, p. 52). This early altered state of consciousness shaped his creative trance in sports and his outlook on life, as seen in his autobiography, *No arms, no legs, no problem: When life happens, you can wish to die or choose to live* (Lujano & Schiro, 2014). After his sports career, Lujano went back to school, obtaining a master's degree in Recreation Sports Management. He is now at the National Center on Health, Physical Activity and Disability in Birmingham, Alabama (Anderson-Maples, 2019).

Paralympic Wheelchair Rugby Team: Achievement and Compassion

Quadriplegic team sports can build a healthy sense of community in their members, ameliorate the isolation that may accompany disability, and generate an acceptance of quadriplegia (Goodwin et al., 2009). With their strengthened connections, a team can act together to benefit society. The medal-winning United States Paralympic wheelchair rugby team, featured in the documentary *Murderball* (Rubin & Shapiro, 2005), helps injured veterans and people in hospital rehabilitation wards adjust to their new lives as disabled individuals. They also interact with children, answering questions about disabilities and demonstrating how they function with wheelchairs. Originally called murderball, wheelchair rugby was designed by quadriplegics for quadriplegics as a fast, aggressive, strategic sport that combines elements of football, ice hockey, and basketball (Goodwin et al., 2009). With all this aggression, there is also compassion.

Blind Visual Artists and the Creative Trance: Esref Armagan

It may seem impossible, but there are totally blind professional visual artists. Two of them are Esref Armagan and Sargy Mann, although there are others. The visual artist Esref Armagan (b. 1953), who was born blind, has had exhibitions of his work (Motluk, 2005; Zausner, 2016). Armagan began drawing as a child by scratching lines that he could feel on cardboard cartons. Now he begins a painting by feeling the object he will represent and then draws his tactile impressions, using pencil on a sheet of paper placed on a rubberized tablet.

The pencil makes depressed lines that his fingers can follow. With the lines as a guide, Armagan uses his fingers to paint, choosing colors that sighted people have told him correspond to objects in the visual world. He has never seen the colors that he places in a specific order for ease of access but selects them from memory to create his works. Armagan is also able to rotate three-dimensional objects in his mind and paint them from different angles, using perspective and shadow.

When a group of neuroscientists studied Armagan (Motluk, 2005), they confirmed he was totally blind. Yet his brain scans indicated that Armagan's visual cortex, which showed activity during his periods of imagination, was even more active while he was painting. It was as if he was seeing. One of the scientists, the neurologist Alvaro Pascual-Leone of Harvard, suggested that although Armagan is without physical vision, his scans indicate the activity of a "mind's eye," which this book would call a creative trance.

Blind Visual Artists and the Creative Trance: Sargy Mann

Another totally blind visual artist with an active mind's eye is the painter Sargy Mann (1937–2015). Although his vision began to fail in his sixties from corneal ulcerations and retinal detachments, Mann continued to create brightly colored canvases (Adams, 2010, n.p.). Painting within his guidelines of moveable Blue Tack putty fragments, Mann vividly sees the color he is painting in his mind's eye. He found that when he used blue, in his mind he saw the canvas turn blue where he was painting. As Mann explains, "The color sensation didn't last, it was only there while I was putting the paint down, but it went on happening with different colors." Mann believes that gradual vision loss was easier for him than sudden blindness, because "my brain kept finding new ways to see the world" (cited in Adams, 2010, n.p.).

The creative trance is so important to artists that they will struggle to maintain it. As Mann says, "Once I had started painting blind, there was no stopping me. It just became the new way of doing it. It was difficult, but art had always been difficult, and having a new set of difficulties was no bad thing" (cited in Adams, 2010, n.p.). That even after vision loss Mann preferred to paint in his usual sunny place outside the studio may have a neurocognitive aspect. Vandewalle and associates (2013) find that light can stimulate cognitive brain activity for some blind individuals who have kept their non-image-forming photoreception.

Blindness and the Haptic Creative Trance: Geerat Vermeij

There are scientific discoveries that can be made without sight because the eyes may overlook what the hands can feel. Haptic perception, which is the capacity to discern objects through touch, is the basis for discoveries made by the paleontologist and evolutionary biologist, Geerat Vermeij (b. 1946). A professor at the University of California at Davis, Vermeij (1997) has been blind since age three when his eyes were removed to eliminate the risk of brain damage due to severe childhood glaucoma.

At age nine, Vermeij had a creative trance that began his scientific career. His family had just moved from the Netherlands to the United States, and in his fourth-grade New Jersey classroom, he felt the beauty of tropical shells for the first time. Unlike the rough chalky shells of Northern Europe, these specimens brought into class from Florida and the Pacific were gleamingly smooth and shiny with domed roofs, fine ribbing, and glossy bead-like protuberances in spiral formations. When his teacher, Mrs. Colberg, spoke about the beaches where the shells were found, Vermeij immediately daydreamed of these exotic places, imagining their warm water and gentle waves depositing beautiful shells on the shore. As Vermeij said (1997, p. 2), "It transformed an ordinary day in the fourth grade" and left him with "a burning curiosity" for the natural world.

Now a leading authority on marine mollusks, Vermeij (1977, 1994) can read shells with their protuberances, damages, and self-repairs as a history of marine life throughout paleontological records. By haptically studying alterations in the architecture of shells, he has been able to elucidate millennia of evolutionary interactions between predator and prey.

Blindness and the Intensity of the Musical Creative Trance

When a great river dividing into tributaries has one of its courses blocked, the river will redirect its flow to other branches. So, it is with sensory abilities. When sight is impaired, hearing may be augmented (Voss et al., 2004) and when hearing is diminished there may be more emphasis on sight (Simon et al., 2020). In sighted people, approximately 85 percent of sensory input to the brain comes from vision (Cytowic, 2018), creating a visually constructed world. Without visual input, the brain can sense the world through hearing and may transform itself to make auditory input the main source of information. A blind person whose world is shaped and interpreted through sound and whose brain has rewired itself to auditory dominance may find that the musical creative trance can assume an enormous importance.

Neuroimaging shows that blindness significantly remaps the brain, which may augment and intensify a musical experience. The brain's cross-modal plasticity allows blind people to use their occipital cortex to process auditory information (Huber et al., 2019). The occipital cortex, which is utilized for vision in the sighted, provides additional brain space for hearing and understanding in the blind. Loiotile and colleagues (2020) found that congenitally blind people who used their occipital cortex to process auditory information outperformed sighted individuals in sentence comprehension.

Blind individuals, especially those with early-onset blindness, can outperform the sighted on a wide range of auditory tasks (Wan et al., 2010). Their enhanced perception of sound includes superior pitch perception and a finer discernment of frequencies (Huber et al., 2019). By relying on information from auditory frequencies for a greater number of activities than sighted people, blind individuals "see" the world with their ears. Ambient sounds encode a rich tapestry of information for the blind (Battalı et al., 2020), and may help to explain how the singer, song writer, and musician Ray Charles (Ray Charles Robinson, 1930–2004) was able to ride a bicycle around his rural Georgia neighborhood without sight as an adventurous child (Ritz & Charles, 2009).

Blindness and the Professional Musical Creative Trance

With their enhanced ability to detect, discriminate, and appreciate sounds, including superior sensitivities to pitch and frequency, it is understandable that blind people have established successful musical careers. Blind individuals who have gained prominence in the eclectic professional music fields of the twentieth to twenty-first centuries include Andrea Bocelli (b. 1958), who sings both classical opera and popular songs, and Jose Feliciano (b. José Monserrate Feliciano García, 1945), a singer, musician, and composer whose work is a fusion of Latin, jazz, blues, and rock. They also include the country music artist "Doc" Watson (b. Arthel Lane Watson, 1923–2012), a guitarist, singer, and songwriter who combined bluegrass, country, gospel music, and blues, and Ronnie Milsap (b. 1943), a singer and musician, combining country and popular music.

In jazz, there is the pianist George Shearing (1919–2011), the singer Diane Schuur (b. 1953), and the singer, songwriter, and musician Jeff Healey (1966–2008), who combined jazz with blues and popular music. These three jazz artists are white, but the greatest percentage of jazz and blues artists who are blind come from the African American community.

Blindness, Medical Care, and the African American Musical Creative Trance

The music of blind African Americans comes from talent nurtured by a music-infused culture. Yet it also comes from poverty and the medical neglect that poverty brings to illnesses that might have been cured in a more affluent setting. In the Appalachian community of the American South, there is also deep poverty and a music-infused culture, but the poverty of the African American community is deeper. In addition, widespread racial prejudice brought an added harshness into their lives. African Americans were often treated very poorly by the medical community, where their symptoms might only be described in medical notes rather than treated as curable conditions (Rowden, 2012).

An example of this type of poor medical care given to African Americans in the South is the U.S. Public Health Service Syphilis Study at Tuskegee (CDC, 2020). This study, begun in 1932, only monitored the progression of syphilis in a group of African American men, but did not tell them why they were included in the experiment. Nor did the study give them penicillin in 1947, when it became known as the most effective medicine to halt the disease. Other illnesses were also inadequately addressed for the African American population, whose home remedies were their most widespread methods of cure.

Medically untreated eye problems significantly increased the number of blind people in the African American community, where blindness was regarded as a hardship rather than a stigma, as it was in certain white communities (Rowden, 2012). Blind individuals were integrated into society and those who were musically gifted were admired and had the possibility of making a professional career. Music was a very viable choice for a talented blind person whose poverty and lack of access to higher education precluded other options.

Early Blindness and Success for African American Music Professionals

In his research on blind African American music professionals, Rowden (2012) finds that almost every blind person with great popular success had either been blind from birth or lost vision at an early age. He suggests that for a blind child, music, with its capacity for regularity, may function as a transitional object to quell the anxiety a child may experience functioning in the sighted world.

In addition, blind children with their enhanced appreciation of sound may have a strong connection to the auditory beauty and power of a musical creative trance. In their world, which is constructed by sound, music is a controlled and ordered sound that can create and shape their experience. Just as drawing brings a sense of self-efficacy to a sighted child, so can making music bring a sense of self-efficacy to a blind child. Music, as a self-generated auditory event, can produce a profound experience of personal power for a blind person. It alters and establishes their world while the music is playing and whenever it is remembered. Music becomes a bridge of creative communication, connecting a personal world to the social world.

Perhaps the most widely known blind African American music professional alive today is Stevie Wonder (Stevland Hardaway Morris, b. 1950). A singer, musician, songwriter, record producer, and activist for humanitarian causes, he was a child prodigy signed to Motown Records at age twelve (Ribowsky, 2010). Wonder lost his sight when as a premature baby he was put into an incubator with an oversupply of oxygen. The hyperoxygenated atmosphere left him with retrolental fibroplasia, which was the leading cause of infant blindness in the 1950s. Wonder gravitated to music at a very early age, and after receiving his first instrument, a harmonica, at age four, he went on to learn multiple instruments. As an adult Wonder pioneered electronic music, blending synthesizers and acoustic sounds, which had a great influence on popular culture.

A Lineage of Blind African American Music Professionals

Stevie Wonder is the modern representative of a long lineage of blind African American music professionals. The individuals cited here are only a partial listing in this lineage of the gifted. Not only are there are other blind African American musicians who have had success, but there are countless individuals with great talent and excellent music who never had an opportunity to record their work or to perform outside of their imme-diate localities. We don't know their names, but it is very possible that their music lives on because they may have influenced the musicians whose names have entered history.

In this lineage, a predecessor to Stevie Wonder is the singer, song writer, and musician Ray Charles (Ray Charles Robinson, 1930–2004). Charles, whose vision gradually diminished to complete blindness at age seven, began losing his sight at age five shortly after witnessing the drowning death of his brother George, age four, in a tub outside their home (Ritz & Charles, 2009). Charles, who felt guilty because he was unable to save his brother, said the tragedy remained so vivid and painful in his memory that it hurt to see it in his mind. Several months after George's death, Charles said his eyes began to make thick mucus tears and his vision started to fade.

At first the nearsightedness only blurred distant horizons but then the myopia increased, and Charles lost sight of nearby objects. Eventually, he could only distinguish night from day. Charles never got an adequate diagnosis for his blindness, but it is possible that it may have been at least partially induced by the trauma of his brother's death. Current research indicates a connection between psychological stress and eye dis-orders (Sabel et al., 2018) with a specific link between childhood trauma and the development of myopia (Katz & Berlin, 2014). Charles, who loved music, started playing the piano at age three, informally taught by his neighbor, Mr. Pitt (Ritz & Charles, 2009). With progressive blindness, the creative trance of music became increasingly important to him.

Later, as a student at the State School for the Blind in St. Augustine, Florida (now the Florida School for the Deaf and the Blind [FSDB]), Charles heard the jazz pianist Art Tatum (Arthur Tatum, Jr., 1909–1956) on the radio and greatly admired his music. Tatum, who lost almost all his sight by age four, became a piano icon, renowned for his unparalleled technical dexterity (Murphy, 2020). This musical lineage also includes the Reverend Gary Davis (1896–1972), a singer and guitarist (Harold & Stone, 2004), Sonny Terry (Saunders Terrell, b. 1911–1986), a singer and harmon-ica player, and the jazz and popular music vocalist Al Hibbler (Albert George Edward Hibbler, 1915–2001) (Rowden, 2012). Hibbler was also an activist in the 1960s civil rights movement.

The Historical Roots of Blind African American Music Professionals

Central to the historical lineage of blind African American music profes-sionals is Blind Lemon Jefferson (Lemon Jefferson, 1893–1929), a Texas singer and guitar player (Monge & Evans, 2003). Believed to be without vision from birth, Jefferson was the first blues singer to make recordings, which widened his musical influence and opened opportunities for other artists. Jefferson's improvisational guitar playing continues to be an inspiration for modern electric blues guitarists. There are also African American groups like the Blind Boys of Alabama, who sing in the gospel tradition and include sighted members.

Another historical recording artist was Blind Blake (Arthur Blake, 1896–1934), who recorded for Paramount (Pace, 1993). Blake was an improvisational ragtime guitar virtuoso and sometimes played with Blind Willie McTell. McTell (William Samuel McTell, 1898–1959), known for his lyrical narratives, lost his sight in childhood, and is honored by the annual Blind Willie McTell Blues Festival in Thompson, Georgia. Unlike the other musicians, Blind Boy Fuller (Fulton Allen, 1903–1941) lost his sight as an adult, at approximately age twenty-four. In response to the illness that was leaving him blind, Fuller increasingly concentrated on his music, possibly to ease his anxiety over continuing vision loss and to earn a living.

The Interstellar Legacy of Blind Willie Johnson

The gospel blues singer and evangelist Blind Willie Johnson (1897–1945) brings us from history to the present and beyond. Johnson, who played slide guitar and piano, went blind at age seven when his stepmother threw lye in his eyes while she was fighting with his father (Blakey, 2016). A religious man, Johnson was a street musician with a tin can hanging from the neck of his guitar whose music was oriented to the spiritual. He recorded for Columbia Records in a makeshift studio set up in a small Atlanta hotel, which greatly increased the influence of his work. In a 1928 recording, Johnson performs a wordless song, *Dark Was the Night – Cold Was the Ground*, on his slide guitar, accompanying the music with an intermittent tuneful moan. Wordless singing has been an established tradition in the religious music of African Americans (Rowden, 2012).

Dark Was the Night – Cold Was the Ground is about the Crucifixion of Jesus, yet as NASA consultant Timothy Ferris said, "Johnson's song concerns a situation he faced many times: nightfall with no place to sleep. Since humans appeared on Earth, the shroud of night has yet to fall without touching a man or woman in the same plight" (cited in NASA, 2020b). In 1977 Johnson's song became one of the twenty-seven pieces of worldwide music placed on NASA's *Voyager Golden Record* and sent into the cosmos on the Voyager probe. Then in 2010 it was added to the

National Recording Registry by the United States Library of Congress (2020), which chooses works considered historically, aesthetically, or culturally significant. Currently, the Voyager probe, with a recording of Johnson's song, continues its journey into deep space (Nelson & Polansky, 1993) with an aim of eventual contact and possibly what this book would consider to be an extraterrestrial audience creative trance.

CHAPTER II

Dementia and the Creative Trance

Survival is not how you end an experience, but how you live through an experience

Dorothy Webb

The desire to create and the endeavor to immortalize a personal conception may overcome even extreme disability

Philip Sandblom

As illness shapes our lives, so can it affect our work, leaving its neural and physiological signatures on our states of creative trance. Sometimes, illness can change life and work for the better (Zausner, 2016), even if it is only for a brief time. This may occur in a wide variety of illnesses and even in the dementias. Although dementia is often associated with the end of a creative life, in its early stages it may allow and even enhance creative work. Dementia's cognitive loss may be feared as a dark night descending on the mind but before nightfall there is sunset, and the creative people in this chapter have magnificent sunset skies filled with all the colors of a sunrise.

Dementia: Its Prevalence and Symptoms

Worldwide, we are an aging population, with dementia affecting people in larger numbers (WHO, 2019). A progressive condition, it creates difficulties with thinking, memory, behavior, and the capacity to perform the activities of everyday life. There are multiple types of dementia: Alzheimer's disease, Lewy body dementia, the frontotemporal dementias, vascular dementia, and mixed dementia, which is the coexistence of at least two forms of dementia.

This chapter will concentrate on two types of dementia: Alzheimer's disease because it is the most prevalent form of dementia, and the primary progressive aphasia (PPA) type of frontotemporal dementia because of its capacity to enhance creativity in music and visual art. While each case of dementia is different and varies according to an individual's personality, the effects of the illness, and the circumstances of care, dementia is categorized by three stages. There is the early stage, where symptoms such as forgetfulness and getting lost gradually appear; the second stage, where symptoms include increased memory lapses and problems with communication and personal care; and the third stage, with symptoms such as an inability to recognize once familiar people, mobility difficulties, and behavioral changes.

Dementia and the Experience of Wholeness in the Creative Trance

Yet despite the continuing brain degradation from dementia that eventually impairs creativity and its creative trance, individuals may not only be creative in the beginning stages of neurological decline but may also fight to remain productive as the illness advances. The sense of wholeness, self-efficacy, and mastery that a creative trance can bring is vital to people with impairments and can be crucial for those facing neurological problems such as dementia. Here, the sense of wholeness encompasses not only making art but also the desire to hold on to the creative self. This is vital in a time of cognitive decline when both the self and the world may feel as if they are slipping away.

For people with a progressive illness, the creative trance is a world apart from the daily world of their illness, where instead of the insurmountable problems of an incurable disease, they face the solvable problems of the creative process. With its connection to the experience of wholeness, a creative trance is at the center of healing modalities across domains and extremely important to individuals with dementia. As a world away from the everyday world, the creative trance is a place of potential and possibilities, seemingly unfettered by the problems of daily existence. In that state, what is not possible in the everyday world exists in its own actuality in the creative trance, bringing feelings of accomplishment that may otherwise seem unavailable. Working despite neurological and physical impairments maintains a creative trance and its sense of a still-empowered self.

Alzheimer's Disease and the Creative Trance: Iris Murdoch

Among the approximately fifty million people worldwide with dementia, 60 to 70 percent have Alzheimer's disease. Neurological markers of this condition include neurofibrillary tangles, senile plaques, synapse loss, and neuroinflammation (Samuel et al., 1994; Bierer et al., 1995; Selkoe, 2002; Heneka et al., 2015). Beginning with memory loss, Alzheimer's disease can include confusion and outbursts of anger, advancing to multiple dysfunctions, and eventually death.

Iris Murdoch (1919–1999) exemplifies determined and continued creativity despite her increasing neurological impairments. A prolific author, she wrote her twenty-sixth and final novel, the 1995 *Jackson's Dilemma*, during the early stages of Alzheimer's disease (Garrard et al., 2004). Although the illness made her creative trance more difficult with diminished cognitive capacities, semantic problems, and repeated bouts of an intense writer's block, Murdoch persevered and finished her book. In their linguistic analysis of the novel, Garrard and associates (2004) find it has a more limited vocabulary, a larger rate of repeated words, and is less syntactically complex than her earlier writing. They attribute her semantic difficulties to a progression of the illness from its early transentorhinal stage to its impairment of the temporal neocortex. Garrard and associates suggest that Murdoch's temporal neocortical problems altered her linguistic capacities.

The 2001 film about Murdoch called *Iris* was based on the book *Elegy for Iris*, written by her husband John Bayley. Bayley (1999, p. 218), who cared for Murdoch during her illness, wrote about his wife's difficulties with the spoken and the written word and described the experience of Alzheimer's disease as "an insidious fog, barely noticeable until everything around has disappeared." Murdoch's previous works were greatly acclaimed, but *Jackson's Dilemma* generated a disappointing critical response. Shortly after its publication, her neurological symptoms worsened until her death in 1999.

That Murdoch was able to complete a novel in the early stages of dementia is a testament to her intellect before the illness and to a lifetime of experience with cognitively demanding work (Garrard et al., 2004). In their data compiled from the Victoria Longitudinal Study, Hultsch and associates (1999) find that high-ability people tend to be intellectually active and that engaging in intellectual activities acts as a protection against cognitive decline in later life. I suggest extending their work to include benefits for all creatively active people, not just intellectually active. It is possible that creativity with its creative trance acts as a strength in the face of advancing cognitive decline.

Alzheimer's Disease and Celebrity Activism: Glen Campbell

Creativity's protective strength is apparent in the life of singer/songwriter Glen Campbell (1936–2017). After his 2011 diagnosis of Alzheimer's disease, until 2014 when he could no longer perform, Campbell made an extended farewell tour, multiple public appearances, a documentary movie, a music video, and released five albums (Selberg, 2017). Despite severe cognitive deficits from the illness, Campbell was able to sing and experience a creative trance because he retained the capacity to carry a melody, although not always in the correct key.

Campbell's accomplishments were supported by a team of professionals, and it was they who shielded his behavioral problems from dementia away from public view. As a celebrity, Campbell raised audience awareness of Alzheimer's disease in what Selberg (2017, pp. 895–896) calls a "heroic battle against loss." Yet he notes that the great majority of individuals with Alzheimer's do not have the wealth and privilege of celebrity status.

Alzheimer's Disease and Celebrity Activism: Rita Hayworth

It was the actor Rita Hayworth (1918–1887) who became the first celebrity face of Alzheimer's disease, although she was misdiagnosed for most of her life. As Lerner (2006) notes, this is because the disease was largely forgotten for over sixty years from the time of its identification in the early twentieth century until the 1970s. He finds that Hayworth's experiences of memory loss were apparent in her fifties. This was also the age of the woman with symptoms of dementia who was presented to Dr. Alois Alzheimer in 1906. Hayworth's outbursts, confusion, and her inability to remember lines eventually halted her acting career. Her last completed film, *The Wrath of God*, was in 1972.

Two years after Hayworth's 1979 diagnosis of Alzheimer's disease, her daughter Princess Yasmin Aga Khan made the diagnosis public. In addition to caring for her mother, Khan became an activist for people with Alzheimer's disease. By increasing public awareness, she wanted to destigmatize the condition and prevent others from being misdiagnosed. Kahn became president of Alzheimer Disease International, and since 1992, the Alzheimer's Association of Chicago has held their Annual Rita Hayworth Gala to promote public acceptance of the illness and raise funds for research.

Alzheimer's disease made life very difficult for Hayworth, who suffered from its extreme mood changes, confusion, and irrational fears. In response, during the early to middle stages of her illness, Hayworth turned to oil painting to express herself and reduce her stress. She produced beautiful paintings with floral imagery. Khan spoke about her mother's positive experience with creativity in a documentary film, *I Remember*

Better When I Paint (Ellena & Huebner, 2009). It demonstrates the beneficial effects of creative arts therapies for people with Alzheimer's disease. She said painting was a way for her mother to calm herself, relax, and find peace of mind. For Hayworth, the creative trance was an emotional haven.

Alzheimer's Disease and Visual Artists

Norman Rockwell's (1894–1978) name also furthers awareness of the illness with the Norman Rockwell Conference on Alzheimer's Disease as a forum for academic research. In the last years of his life, Rockwell was unable to paint because of advancing dementia (Claridge, 2001). Alzheimer's disease may impede the creation of visual art by producing more simplified works, altering perspective, having fewer angles, and impairing spatial relations (Kirk & Kertesz, 1991). Although the illness leaves neurological damage in both brain hemispheres, drawing ability is associated with right hemisphere and degeneration of the right hemisphere, which processes visuospatial information, can be an early aspect of Alzheimer's disease (Meulenberg, 1996; Miller et al., 2005).

Despite their continuing neurological impediments from Alzheimer's disease, two classically trained professional visual artists, the abstract painter Willem de Kooning and the figurative painter William Utermohlen, struggled to remain creative. In a time of cognitive impairment, creativity and its creative trance can be an island of solidity, a semblance of clarity in an encroaching fog of dementia. As a result of their efforts, each in their own way succeeded in creating original works during the illness.

Alzheimer's Disease and Willem de Kooning

At times dementia prevented Willem de Kooning (1904–1997) from distinguishing between his wife and his sister, yet he fought to remain creative, insisting, "I paint to live!" (cited in Espinel, 1996, p. 1097). Like many creative people, de Kooning felt most alive when he was working, but in dementia, his creative trance took on an increasing urgency. It helped him retain his semblance of self, becoming a rock of refuge in an increasingly amorphous and dissolving world. In the last decade of his life, when he could no longer sign his name, de Kooning could still function in his creative trance, working at his easel, or sitting and assessing a canvas in progress (Kontos, 2003).

This drive to maintain himself through self-expression produced his late works in the 1980s and created a new style. Although aspects of the late paintings were based on his earlier canvases, de Kooning would rework them, often letting his hand with its brush roam freely, unfettered by his conscious mind (Espinel, 1996). While artists can create with cognitive discernment, they can also paint with their embodied knowledge of skills, which is their implicit or procedural memories of making brushstrokes. It is possible that the large curvilinear forms in de Kooning's late works may have been created in this way (Kontos, 2003; Espinel, 2007).

Willem de Kooning: Alzheimer's Disease, Mixed Dementia, and Continued Creativity

In addition to Alzheimer's disease, de Kooning's dementia may also have its origins in alcoholism, arteriosclerosis, Korsakoff's syndrome, which is a type of alcohol-related dementia, and overuse of prescription drugs (Espinel, 1996). In the 1970s, depressed, alcoholic, and over reliant on prescription medications, with a history of self-neglect and poor nutrition, de Kooning began showing signs of cognitive difficulties, and had ceased to paint. With care from his wife Elaine and a group of friends, de Kooning stopped drinking, ate well, exercised, received medical attention, went to psychotherapy, and joined Alcoholics Anonymous (Stewart, 2002; Kontos, 2003). Two years later, after regaining his strength, and despite advancing dementia, he returned to his studio.

De Kooning began to paint again, this time with an electric easel that rotated his canvases, and the help of studio assistants. Alzheimer's disease influenced his creative trance and altered his late works by reducing their complexity, limiting their color palette, and flattening their compositions relative to his earlier paintings. Yet their graceful arcs of paint in curvilinear abstract forms are well positioned on the white backgrounds. Although there was a negative critical response to the late works (Meulenberg, 1996), Stewart (2002, p. 319) believes we should focus on Kooning's perseverance and his creativity, saying, "Do we, in this society, classify a person by what he has lost, or rather, what he has accomplished in spite of that loss."

Alzheimer's Disease and William Utermohlen

In 1991, when William Utermohlen (1933–2007) was age fifty-seven, he had noticeable memory impairments, problems with words, and could not easily tell the time nor find his way home. His symptoms kept increasing in severity and in 1995 Utermohlen was diagnosed with Alzheimer's disease. Neurological tests showed global cognitive deterioration with pronounced cerebral atrophy (Crutch et al., 2001; Pollini, 2014). Upon learning about this diagnosis, his wife said Utermohlen "began to paint himself, desperately trying to understand what was happening to his mind" (Utermohlen, 2006,).

In response to the illness, Utermohlen made a series of self-portraits to maintain his sense of self, despite the relentless progression of the disease. These self-portraits were his concrete markers in a dissolving world and have become some of the most widely cited works of art charting cognitive decline due to Alzheimer's disease.

For Utermohlen, as it was for de Kooning, the creative trance brought a sense of self-efficacy and control that was quickly eroding in other aspects of life. In 1996, the first self-portrait after Utermohlen's diagnosis is a realistically painted but flattened and yellowed face, showing his features pulled into a grimace by the illness and his stress. As the self-portraits continue from 1996 until 2000, they decline in recognizability as his dementia advances. The very last images barely resemble a face at all. In their *Lancet* article on Utermohlen's work and his illness, Crutch and associates (2001, p. 2133) call the artist's perseverance despite inexorable neurological decline "a testament to the resilience of human creativity."

William Utermohlen: The Positive Effects of Alzheimer's Disease on His Art

Yet toward the beginning of Utermohlen's illness, Alzheimer's disease influenced his creative trance in a very positive way. It was during that brief window of time when his vision was already altered but his cognitive problems were not yet severe that Utermohlen experienced enhanced creativity from Alzheimer's disease. From 1990 to 1991, he made six very large vibrantly colored oil paintings called the *Conversation Pieces*, images of the artist, his wife, and their friends at his home.

Although the paintings show conversations, the images of verbal interactions are most often portraits of his wife and friends, not of the artist. In one painting five people sit around a table talking, while Utermohlen shows himself off to the side, sitting on a couch and holding a cat. It suggests that even though he could make wonderful works of visual art, verbal interaction had become difficult for him, and he was self-isolating with a comforting nonverbal feline companion. In these paintings, with their flattened perspective, intensely slanted Escher-like spatial planes, upended tables, and tilting chairs, Utermohlen uses the visual distortions of Alzheimer's disease to bring a vibrant intensity to his work.

The dramatic effects in Utermohlen's paintings are possible because in the beginning stages of Alzheimer's disease, there can be damage to the visual cortex, which alters visuospatial perceptions (Meulenberg, 1996; Miller et al., 2005). This change may occur before memory impairment is evident, as it did with Utermohlen (Butter et al., 1996; Possin, 2010). It suggests there might have been less hippocampal decline at that time, which would leave the capacity for memory. Concurrently, there was also a possible increased atrophy of the occipital and parietal cortex, areas of the brain that work with visuospatial information. These neurological impairments structured Utermohlen's creative trance by altering his spatial perception. This may have facilitated the extremely dramatic compositions and flattened patterns that form the basis of his excellent and original art.

Dementia and Creativity: The Transforming Illness and Paradoxical Functional Facilitation

Cognitive decline is often but not always accompanied by a loss of creativity. Yet as we see with William Utermohlen, in some instances, especially in the early phases of the illness, dementia may restructure and enhance the creative trance. When this happens, the influence of illness may be so profound that it becomes a turning point in the creative process. Then I would call it a *transforming illness* (Zausner, 2016) because it transforms the work produced, turning problems into pathways.

Dementia may augment creativity in an additional way, yet again for only a limited time. Called paradoxical functional facilitation (Kapur, 1996), it occurs when the results of neural damage enhance behavioral functioning. These new abilities emerging during dementia appear to indicate that a loss of capacity in one area of the brain may enhance capabilities elsewhere. This type of facilitation can occur in in frontotemporal dementia (FTD). In FTD, impaired verbal functioning in the left hemisphere of the brain may give more prominence to the right hemisphere, enhancing the creation of music and visual art. This alteration in prominence affected the life and work of the composer Maurice Ravel and the visual artist Anne Theresa Adams.

Frontotemporal Dementia and Creativity

Frontotemporal dementia is a neurodegenerative illness that generally has an earlier onset than Alzheimer's disease. Yet despite its progressive brain damage, there are instances when FTD profoundly enhances visual and musical creativity (Miller et al., 1998; Miller et al., 2000; Miller & Hou, 2004). This can occur in a type of FTD called primary progressive aphasia (PPA), which is a semantic dementia where words eventually become unattainable. In FTD, the left anterior temporal lobe, which is involved in language processing, functions at a permanently low metabolic rate, possibly allowing the right hemisphere and its creative capacities to come forward (Amaducci et al., 2002; Miller & Hou, 2004; Seeley et al., 2008). When Miller and associates (2000) tested a group of patients with the PPA type of FTD at the University of California, San Francisco, Memory and Aging Center, they found that those who showed a greater loss of verbal function were the ones who kept and even advanced their visual or musical skills.

When individuals develop FTD, it alters their creativity and, in doing so, appears to generate a similar structure to their creative trance in music and art. They may have a compulsive aspect to their creativity, feel driven to create, producing works with bold elements of style, arranged in pronounced patterns of repetition, and in visual art they tend to use brighter colors (Miller & Hou, 2004). Perhaps these strong organizing aspects become an anchor of strength, an assuaging counterpoint to the loss of semantic abilities in an increasingly difficult cognitive environment. Examples of FTD musical creativity would be the dramatic late works of Maurice Ravel, and in visual art, it is the paintings of Anne Theresa Adams.

Frontotemporal Dementia and Maurice Ravel

The composer Maurice Ravel (1875–1937) is perhaps the most well-known creative person diagnosed with the PPA type of FTD (Seeley et al., 2008). By 1927, Ravel had begun to exhibit language problems, and by 1932, he had difficulties with speaking, reading, writing, and forming words (aphasia, alexia, agraphia, and apraxia) (Henson, 1988; Amaducci et al., 2002; Cavallera et al., 2012). Yet during that window of time, he showed a great ability for musical creativity. Then in 1932, Ravel's problems worsened after a head trauma from a traffic accident aggravated his underlying neurological condition. Words became increasingly difficult for Ravel and then almost impossible, which was an extreme frustration. Eventually he could not sign his name and after 1932, he could no longer transcribe his music into words.

This was a great hardship for Ravel. He was planning to write an opera and while he could hear the music in his mind, he could not write it on paper. There was a musically intact, unwritten opera, still vibrant in his creative trance. Yet because he could not transcribe it, the music remained forever unshared. As he confided to a friend in 1933, "I will never write my *Jeanne d'Arc*; this opera is here, in my head, I hear it, but I will never write it. It's over, I can no longer write my music" (cited in Amaducci et al., 2002, p. 76). Coordination problems from advancing FTD eventually made piano playing no longer possible, nor was he able conduct an orchestra (Henson, 1988). Ravel died in 1937 after a surgery that unsuccessfully attempted to address his illness.

Frontotemporal Dementia: Maurice Ravel's *Bolero* and Later Works

Yet aphasia, which is the loss of language capacities, does not mean there is also amusia, the loss of musical abilities. During the appearance of clinical symptoms in 1928, Ravel composed *Bolero*, his most famous work (Amaducci et al., 2002; Seeley et al., 2008). Originally intended as a ballet, it was danced by Ida Rubinstein, Ravel's lifelong friend. *Bolero* appears to derive its structure and power from the influence of FTD with its repeating musical forms, intensifying volume, staccato drums, and escalating number of instruments. The music was enormously successful starting with its debut at the Paris Opera House to its continuing popularity today.

Ravel's illness continued to progress, further altering the balance between his brain hemispheres and affecting his creative trance. Amaducci, Grassi, and Boller (2002) find that a later work, the 1929 to 1930 *Piano Concerto for the Left Hand*, increasingly suggests the influence of FTD with its shorter less elaborate phrasing, its pulsating irregular style with syncopation and tempo changes, and its great range of timbres. The concerto was commissioned by Paul Wittgenstein, a pianist who lost his right arm in World War I. Wittgenstein, brother of the philosopher Ludwig Wittgenstein, also gave the concerto's initial performance in Vienna, 1931. For Wittgenstein, the creative trance was playing the piano and performing. Denied this by most works for the piano, Wittgenstein also commissioned piano pieces for the left hand from Hindemith, Britten, Richard Strauss, and Prokofiev.

When the contemporary pianist Andre Watts (b. 1946) had nerve damage in his left hand, he transcribed Ravel's concerto to be played by the right hand (Gubar, 2020) but unfortunately the concerts where he was scheduled to perform were canceled due to the coronavirus. In 1931, Ravel completed another work, the *G-Major Concerto*, but Amaducci, Grassi, and Boller (2002) believe it was based on music predating his illness and does not exhibit the right hemispheric influences shown in the *Piano Concerto for the Left Hand* and in the *Bolero*.

Frontotemporal Dementia and Anne Theresa Adams

Anne Theresa Adams (1940–2007), who also developed the PPA type of FTD, had a fascination with Ravel's *Bolero* and made it the subject of her most widely cited painting, the 1994 diptych *Unravelling Bolero* (Seeley et al., 2008). In this work, Adams translates Ravel's music into visual form, using colors and shapes that she associates with individual musical notes. Ravel's music, structured by FTD, resonated with Adams across domains because her creative trance and its resulting work were shaped by the same illness. It appears that Adams recognized this affinity. She presented her doctors with a scientific article on Ravel's neurological condition and noted its similarity to her own.

Adams, a scientist with a PhD in cell biology, held university research and teaching positions, and although she was interested in visual art since childhood, it was just a hobby. Then in 1986, her son was gravely injured in an auto accident. When it appeared that he might need years of intensive treatment, Adams stopped her academic work to care for him. While at home with her son, Adams, turned to art, possibly for a calming creative trance in a very difficult time. Creativity, with its capacity for mood repair, its ability to increase life satisfaction, and its orientation toward personal growth (Futterman Collier & Wayment, 2021), brought about a significant change in Adams' life.

When her son made an incredible recovery within two months, Adams decided to permanently leave her biomedical research at the university and become a full-time visual artist. Her profound career change may also have been a result of post-traumatic growth (Taylor, 2012; Rendon, 2015), generated by the trauma of seeing her son severely injured. Trauma can inspire an internal reorganization, possibly by revealing a previously neglected aspect of life, recognizing its importance, and bringing it forward, as Adams did with her art.

Anne Theresa Adams: The Positive Effects of Frontotemporal Dementia on Her Art

Before the onset of FTD, Adams painted competent realistic works. Yet by 1993, the illness had altered her art for the better by dramatically emphasizing patterns, colors, and repeated shapes that structure and strengthen her compositions (Zausner, 2016). While the effects of FTD on Adams' creative trance and her art predated the appearance of clinical symptoms in 2000, a 1997 MRI to monitor an acoustic neuroma showed that degeneration in areas of the frontal cortex associated with language processing had already begun (Seeley et al., 2008). This indicates that visual creativity can emerge and progress despite ongoing left hemisphere deterioration.

Highly focused on creativity, Adams spent most of her waking hours making art. In addition to *Unravelling Bolero*, she created visual interpretations of other pieces of music including Gershwin's *Rhapsody in Blue* (Seeley et al., 2008). Like *Bolero, Rhapsody in Blue* is dramatic, with great orchestral color, pronounced rhythm, and clear musical repetitions. Adams also produced *pi*, a visual translation of the first 1,471 digits of the bounded infinite decimal pi (π), and interpreted her migraine as a geometrical design. She created hyper-realistic images of natural objects, such as stones, and made a series of works, the *ABC Book of Invertebrates*, where the animals are all listed alphabetically and shown as repeating patterns in mandala-like circular designs.

These are all excellent strong, original works, but as the FTD progressed, Adams returned to competent realistic scenes. Although her mental and physical capacities were waning, creativity with its creative trance imparted a sense of wholeness and self-efficacy to Adams as it does to so many creative people. In response, and despite her illness, Adams persisted in painting until she could no longer hold a brush.

Frontotemporal Dementia: Neuroplasticity and Acquired Savant Capacities

Our brains, ever malleable, are continually changing in response to experience, and it is possible that both Adams' illness and her perseverance in creativity stimulated neuroplasticity that improved her work. It is not uncommon for visual artists to spend long hours in the studio, but for Adams, the compulsive aspect of her illness may have augmented this tendency, while increasing her artistic abilities through repeated practice. Creativity can be compulsive for people with FTD, who may become perfectionists, repeating their work, and improving their abilities (Miller & Hou, 2004). Just as London taxi drivers with extensive navigation knowledge of London streets have significantly larger posterior hippocampi (Maguire et al., 2000), it is possible that Adams' extreme focus on work also facilitated brain changes.

Using neuroimaging, Seeley and associates (2008) suggest that Adams' left hemisphere damage liberated her right hemisphere to assume a greater role. Specifically, they found that despite the continuing FTD impairment to her language processing capacities in the left inferior temporal cortex, Adams added extra gray matter tissue to her healthy right posterior neocortex. The new structural and functional enhancements to her right posterior neocortex may have increased Adams' capacity for visual creativity and presumably enhanced her creative trance. Adams' brain augmentation is an example of positive neuroplasticity in the face of neurological decline.

Bruce Miller (2006), Director of the University of California, San Francisco, Memory and Aging Center, believes Adams' abilities are so extraordinary that they suggest acquired savant capacities. He says that loss of brain tissue from FTD permits other areas of the brain to become more active, transforming an individual from a generalist to a specialist, with specialized capabilities like those of a savant. Adams went from painting competent works of art before her illness to painting works of extraordinary originality during her illness. These works required not only exceptional drawing skills but also original thinking. Even in dementia our brains can evolve, and our states of creative trance can evolve, and our work can attain new levels of excellence.

CHAPTER 12

Altered States of a Lifesaving Creative Trance

True inspiration overrides all fears. When you are inspired, you enter a trance state and can accomplish things that you may never have felt capable of doing

Bernie Siegel

To save one life is to save the world

The Talmud and the Quran

Creativity and its trance states permeate our lives, from the inner musings of daily decisions to lifesaving acts of heroism that far exceed ordinary human limitations. The range of these altered states reflects our extensive capabilities as human beings. Altered states of a creative trance were pivotal to Robert Wagner "Wag" Dodge, who invented a new way to reroute the path of flames in the middle of a raging forest fire.

Altered states also occur in response to the urgent need to save a life when individuals lift a multi-thousand-pound vehicle to rescue a person trapped beneath it. The rescue appears to be impossible, yet the individuals succeed by using abilities seemingly beyond normal comprehension. They display a power anecdotally called *hysterical strength*, which this book calls *extraordinary human strength* (EHS). This capacity, which manifests infrequently and only in certain people, arises in response to the critical need to save a life. With its enormous power, its focused yet open mind, its creative strategic problem-solving, and its altered states of consciousness, extraordinary human strength is an apex in the evolution of the everyday creative trance. It demonstrates that in specific circumstances, we may have access to greater capacities than we realize and far exceed the presumed limits of human beings.

Crisis and the Lifesaving Creative Trance: Wag Dodge

While the creativity of eminent individuals can alter the course of civilizations, certain instances of everyday creativity may be the most individually

174

dramatic. In times of great necessity, the everyday problem-solving trance can escalate into lifesaving heroism that ensures the safety of following generations. This happened when the firefighter Robert Wagner "Wag" Dodge (1915–1955) discovered a new way to control the path of a rapidly advancing forest fire in a Montana national park.

It was 12:25 in the afternoon of August 5, 1949, when reports came in about a wildfire started by lightning in the Mann Gulch area of Helena National Forest (Maclean, 2017; Rothermel, 1993; Alexander et al., 2009; Kounios & Beeman, 2015). There were no roads to the location, so a team of fifteen smokejumpers, firefighters parachuting from a C-47 plane, were sent to fight the blaze. At Mann Gulch, the smokejumpers met with a fire guard from a nearby area. Of these sixteen individuals, only three would survive. Shortly after the men arrived, a heavy wind picked up, and what was initially reported as a routine fire exploded into a blowup with whirling vortices, which are whirlwinds of fire.

The team foreman, Wag Dodge, an intuitive man given to long silences, was unnerved by the blaze. Even before the wind came up, he called it a deathtrap. To keep his team safe, he steered them toward the river and when the wind pushed the fire forward, he told his men to drop their equipment for an unencumbered flight to safety. Now with the flames coming faster than a man could run up the steep slope of the almost vertical gulch, Dodge stopped, paused, and turned inwards. Using a creative trance state to establish a boundary from the crisis, he was able to calculate the variables more efficiently. Gaining insight about how to redirect the blaze, he calmly took out a matchbook and lit a fire in the tall grass in front of him, directly in the path of the oncoming flames.

Insight in Crisis and the Lifesaving Creative Trance: Wag Dodge

It was his idea that a swath of embers would steer the flames around and away from the burnt area and it did. Dodge called out his men to join him in the refuge of burnt ground, but they thought he was crazy and tried in vain to outrun the flames. "For all my hollering," Dodge later reported, "I could not direct anyone into the burnt area" (cited in Maclean, 2004, p. 23). Two men who survived by climbing through a crevice in the rock wall and finding refuge in a rockslide admitted that they thought Dodge's idea was insane at the time. The other thirteen perished in the flames.

Dodge's inspiration during a crisis-generated creative trance is now known as an escape fire and has become a staple of firefighting instruction (Alexander et al., 2009). Waiting out the ten-foot-tall flames face down on burnt ground was not easy for Dodge, who was lifted into the air three times by the convection updrafts of the conflagration. Escape fires were used by the Native American tribes in the area, but they were not yet known to firefighters before Dodge's actions in Mann Gulch. Although Dodge was not able to rescue the thirteen men who perished in 1949, escape fires have saved many lives since then.

The Neuroscience of Insight and Analysis

Citing their research on the neuroscience of insight, Kounios and Beeman (2015) believe Dodge's decision infers activity in the anterior cingulate and the temporal lobes of the brain. They say this because Dodge came to the unusual consideration of fighting fire with fire, and not an immediate first choice of running away. Kounios and Beeman refer to fMRI imaging of brains during insight showing activity in the anterior cingulate and the temporal lobes. They suggest that the anterior cingulate monitors other brain regions for competing solutions to a problem. When the anterior cingulate is active, we become open to a wider range of possible solutions, even those that are not immediately obvious. They describe these as outlier ideas waiting in the temporal lobes. Dodge entered a creative trance during his crisis, and an open searching brain addressing multiple variables is a hallmark of its dynamics.

Conversely when the anterior cingulate is not active, we tend to have an analytic mindset. Kounios and Beeman (2015, p. 91) note that during analytic problem-solving there is widespread activation of the visual areas of the brain, suggesting "seeing" solutions through visualization. Because visualization is an aspect of the creative trance, we may infer that both analytical and intuitive problem-solving have their states of trance. Some problems may call for both modes. Wag Dodge may have initiated his problem-solving through intuitive ideas such as fighting fire with fire but then used the analytical mode to calculate the size and position of the lifesaving patch of burnt ground.

Crisis and the Lifesaving Creative Trance: Extraordinary Human Strength

Another type of lifesaving creative trance is the dramatic rescue using extraordinary human strength. Its most common occurrence is the seemingly impossible action of one individual lifting a car to free another person trapped beneath it. This heroic feat, inspired by extreme emotion, leads to instant action without rumination, and appears to occur in an altered state of consciousness. Coming from an urgent and profound concern for the person in distress, it combines with a desire to rescue that person and immediately alleviate the suffering.

The entire focus is on the other person, who is in great danger. There appears to be no thoughts for oneself or one's own condition, needs, vulnerability to injury, or any awareness of personal limitations. The experience incorporates unusual capacities, which may include exceeding the normal range of human physical strength, a lack of logically assessing that the rescue may be impossible, along with elements of dissociation. Anecdotally linked with the possible release of natural stimulants produced by the body such as adrenaline, norepinephrine (noradrenaline), and cortisol, these experiences are not currently documented in the scientific literature. Arising without warning, they cannot be ethically reproduced in laboratory settings due to their inherent danger. Yet, perhaps if simulated through virtual reality, rescue efforts may at some point be more amenable to quantified research.

Another difficulty for quantified measurement is that the people who have experienced extraordinary human strength do not appear to be able to summon it on command. When Marie "Bootsy" Payton's granddaughter was pinned beneath her riding lawnmower, Payton grabbed the machine and easily tossed it away, freeing the child (Clark, 2019). Yet later, when there was no child to save and Payton tried to lift the lawnmower again, she could not even move it. Tom Boyle, Jr., lifted a three-thousand-pound Camaro car to free a man and his bicycle trapped beneath it, yet in an interview about his heroism, Boyle said, "There's no way I could lift that car right now" (cited in Wise, 2009a, p. 27).

Extraordinary Human Strength as Inspiration for the *Hulk*

Although instances of extraordinary human strength are not yet in academic journals, they are recorded in the media with substantiating witness accounts and have influenced popular culture. In an interview, the comic book writer and artist Jack Kirby (1917–1994) said a Marvel Comics superhero that he created with Stan Lee was inspired by viewing an incident of extraordinary human strength (Groth, 2011). Kirby revealed that his idea for the *Hulk*, who transforms through extreme emotion from the reclusive scientist Dr. Robert Bruce Banner into the large powerful green Hulk, came from the time he witnessed a mother lifting a car to free her child caught beneath it.

The child had been playing in the street when he became trapped under the running board of a car as he tried to crawl up to the sidewalk. Seeing her endangered child, the distraught mother lifted the rear end of the vehicle to save him. Kirby said (cited in Groth, 2011, online), "This woman proved to me that the ordinary person in desperate circumstances can transcend himself and do things that he wouldn't ordinarily do."

Crisis and the Lifesaving Creative Trance: Charlotte Heffelmire and Lauren Kornacki

Kirby's observation that in desperate circumstances people can perform extraordinary acts of heroism applies to two women, Charlotte Heffelmire and Lauren Kornacki, who lifted heavy vehicles to free their fathers. Coincidentally, both women lived in the state of Virginia, USA, but are chosen as examples because of the degree of substantiating evidence validating their EHS events. Both spoke online about their experiences, received extensive media coverage, with reliable witness corroboration, had medical records, and confirmations by a government agency, the Fairfax County Fire Department, and a nonprofit organization, the American Heart Association.

Charlotte Heffelmire: EHS and the Lifesaving Creative Trance

Charlotte Heffelmire (b. 1996) was age nineteen and a student at the United States Air Force Academy when she was home from school during her Thanksgiving break (Fox, 2016; Mann, 2016; NBC4 News, 2016; Haseltine, 2018). On November 26, 2016, she entered the garage of her family home in Vienna, Virginia, and saw her father, Eric Heffelmire, pinned underneath his burning GMC utility pickup truck. He had been working on its brake lines and had a wheel removed when the jack slipped, pinning him underneath the vehicle, while the leaking gasoline started a fire. Despite the fire and smoke, the barefoot five-foot-six-inch 120-pound Heffelmire lifted the pickup truck by its fender twice, rested the empty wheel hub on her hip, and pulled her father out from under it to safety.

Then, not wanting the house to explode because of the burning truck, she put it into four-wheel drive and drove the three-wheeled pickup truck out of the garage. Returning to the house, Heffelmire closed the garage door to contain the flames, got the rest of her family to safety, and calmly called 911, which is the emergency number in the United States. Heffelmire, who received the Citizen Lifesaving Award from the Fairfax

County Fire Department, insists she is not a hero, but only someone doing what was necessary.

Lauren Kornacki: EHS and the Lifesaving Creative Trance

In the summer of 2012, Lauren Kornacki (b. 1989) was a recent graduate of the University of Mary Washington with a major in physics, and living at home in Glen Allen, Virginia (CNN Wire Staff, 2012; Newcomb, 2012; American Heart Association News Archive, 2014; Jung, 2019). She was working as the manager of a local pool when she came home to find her father, Alex Kornacki, in the family garage. He was pinned under his 1995 BMW, with his arm over his chest, unconscious and unresponsive. Alex Kornacki had been changing the brake pads on the right-side rear tire when the jack gave way, trapping him underneath the car.

Kornacki called to her mother and sister, who were home at the time, to dial 911. Then, placing her hand underneath the fender she lifted the vehicle and pulled her father free. When Kornacki started CPR chest compressions, her father began breathing again. The ambulance came and took Alex Kornacki to Virginia Commonwealth University Medical Center where he was treated for multiple fractures and numbness in his arm but made an excellent recovery. Commended by the American Heart Association for using CPR, Kornacki says she doesn't consider herself to be a hero, nor does she compare herself to the Hulk.

Extraordinary Human Strength: Strategic Problem-Solving Creativity

For both Heffelmire and Kornacki, selfless love and devotion became heightened in response to an extreme crisis. They appeared to engage in actions without cognitive reflection as to whether the rescue would be possible, yet with excellent problem-solving activity. Their strategic actions were a creative response that mitigated a life-or-death crisis in daily living, suggesting the experience of a lifesaving creative trance.

Each woman was highly strategic in responding to the needs of her specific emergency and the order in which her actions were accomplished. Upon entering the garage and seeing her unconscious father pinned under his car, Kornacki immediately called to her mother and sister to dial 911, then picked up the car, pulled her unconscious father out, and began CPR. Heffelmire entered a burning garage barefoot, realized the danger of an imminent explosion, but did not run back into the house for shoes. Instead, she lifted the pickup truck twice, freed her father, and drove the burning three-wheeled truck out of the garage so the house would not catch fire from an explosion. Then after making sure her family was safe, she dialed 911.

Extraordinary Human Strength as an Altered State of Consciousness

Both Heffelmire and Kornacki lifted a vehicle weighing thousands of pounds off a beloved father with no thoughts that it might be impossible or that they could be injured. In addition, after initially lifting the vehicle, both women pulled a grown man out from under it. An initial indication that the experience appears to occur in an altered state of consciousness is that neither woman experienced the vehicle as heavy. "I didn't feel like I was lifting anything," said Heffelmire. "I just felt like I was lifting a piece of paper" (cited in Fox, 2016 [video file]). Kornacki stated, "I just literally lifted up the car. It was like a table with a short leg. It kind of balanced back out and shifted enough to free my dad" (cited in Newcomb, 2012, online). Another indication that the women were in an altered state of consciousness is that neither woman reported she engaged in logical reasoning, such as the vehicle might be too heavy to lift or that she could endanger herself. Instead, they were emotion-driven to save a loved one.

Heffelmire said she could not fully explain the experience. "I just freaked out at that moment . . . I had this crazy strength" (cited in Fox, 2016 [video file]). Her trance state appears to have started before discovering her father in distress. "I had the feeling that something was weird," Heffelmire stated, "so I opened the garage door, and the entire garage was black" (cited in DeGeneres, 2016 [video file]). Then she heard her father say, "You have to lift the truck." Coming into the garage she saw, it "was already on fire and really from there I kind of snapped into whatever super mode I had at that point and kind of did what I had to do" (cited in Mann, 2016).

Extraordinary Human Strength: Dissociative Aspects

Evidence suggests the presence of dissociative aspects in the experiences of both women. Although Heffelmire was barefoot all the time she entered the burning garage, lifted the car, pulled her father out, and then drove the burning truck away, she did not report feeling any pain during her life-saving actions. Yet after the event, burns to her feet and hands, along with a back injury, interrupted her studies at the Air Force Academy. When asked about her future, Heffelmire said, "Right now I'm just healing up and making sure the family is OK" (cited in NBC4 News, 2016).

Although Kornacki revealed that the experience was terrifying for her, she did not stop to think before saving her father, explaining her actions as "Everyone has a basic instinct to help the ones they love" (cited in Jung, 2019). "All I could think was my dad wasn't OK," said Kornacki. "I just knew I had to get him out of harm's way." When she called to her mother and sister to dial 911, her mother later described it as a primal scream. Kornacki does not remember what she was thinking. Her only focus was on saving her father with no thoughts that it might be impossible.

EHS: Emotion, Cognition, Peptides, and the Fear Response

Both Heffelmire and Kornacki were under great pressure to save their fathers, and each woman was profoundly afraid that her father might die. Wise (2009a, 2009b), who associates EHS with the experience of extreme fear, believes that the body's fear response unleashes stores of energy that in normal circumstances would remain inaccessible. He describes this as a full activation of the hypothalamic-pituitary-adrenaline axis and the sympathetic nervous system, which make their resources available under the acute stress of fear. The sympathetic nervous system readies the body for continued, energetic action while the adrenal glands release adrenaline and cortisol to the bloodstream. The heart rate increases and blood pressure elevates, supplying the muscles with energy and oxygen. Yet the extreme fear Heffelmire and Kornacki experienced was not a fear for their own welfare but a compassionate fear for the well-being of a loved one.

Heffelmire and Kornacki were able to respond immediately both physically and emotionally without cognitive reflection because we have evolved that way to save our lives and the lives of others. It is a survival instinct. Emotional responses are faster than cognitive thought because the limbic system, which is the emotional center of the brain, sends out alerts before the rational part of the brain can process an event (Sterrett, 2014). In response we are prepared to act immediately, empowered by the emotional response flooding our bodies.

Pharmacological research (Pert et al., 1985; Pert, 1997) indicates that emotions are a bodywide biochemical event generated by an extensive system of peptides and receptors. This network, densest in the limbic area of the brain, extends into the glands and the immune system, making emotions a widespread physical experience. Perhaps the extreme emotional response generated by Heffelmire and Kornacki, carried by peptides to receptors throughout the body, combined with great fear and profound selflessness created a condition that became an entryway to access the enormous strength necessary for the rescue.

Extraordinary Human Strength: The Dorsal System and the Ventral System

Another possible reason that the women assumed they were physically able to lift a multi-thousand-pound vehicle is that in their emotion-driven altered state, they appeared to have no conscious awareness that it might be logically impossible or dangerous. They acted immediately out of love and panic without stopping for reflection. A suggested explanation for their actions is that information can reach our brain and generate a physical response without forming the words for conscious deliberation. Cognitive neuroscience finds there are two different and independently functioning visual input pathways in the brain, the dorsal system and the ventral system (Goodale & Milner, 1992; Goodale & Westwood, 2004). Both systems start in the striate cortex, with the ventral stream going to the inferotemporal cortex and the dorsal stream going to the posterior parietal region.

Each system uses its visual input from the world in a different way. The dorsal stream controls visually guided action, usually processing its information without conscious awareness, while the ventral stream, which is generally available to consciousness, processes perception and recognition. Although the systems can engage in crosstalk, it is possible for one system to dominate, and during extraordinary human strength, it appears to be the dorsal system. As Bargh (2005, p. 45) states, the dorsal stream with its nonconscious action could "drive behavior in response to environmental stimuli in the absence of conscious awareness or understanding of that external information." While Bargh connects dorsal activation with mirror neurons and nonconscious imitative motor movements, the emotional component of mirror neuron activity may be an aspect of extraordinary human strength. By internally mirroring the life-threatening situation of a loved one, mirror neurons may enhance the motivation to rescue.

EHS: Naturally Occurring Stimulants and Possible Unmeasured Forces

Research on the effects of naturally occurring stimulants such as adrenaline, norepinephrine (noradrenaline), and cortisol in sports, exercise, and hand grip indicate they are associated with strength that can increase during a time of challenge (Pratley et al., 1994; Davis et al., 2008; Ribeiro et al., 2016). Yet all the strength measurements in the research studies were well within the normal human range. A defining aspect of extraordinary human strength is its beyond-normal range of physical capacity, so there appear to be other factors involved.

The difference in capacity between the measurements of strength in research studies and the extreme power of extraordinary human strength suggests that in the latter, there may be yet unmeasured forces at work. Currently, there is no definitive explanation for the appearance of beyond-normal strength or the energy source for this rare and dramatic type of creative trance. In response, the remainder of the chapter will investigate conceivable explanations for the phenomena, beginning with clinical aspects and continuing to multiple possibilities in Eastern philosophies and contemporary physics.

Extraordinary Human Strength: Clinical Aspects

The words and actions of Heffelmire and Kornacki suggest that their experiences of extraordinary human strength took place in an altered state of consciousness. Their actions were generated by profound emotional investment and the desire to help with no thoughts of self-welfare. Clinical analysis of their lifesaving actions during the rescue suggests a completely other-centered focus of mind, a close relationship with the father, and when commended for their bravery, there was no sign of narcissistic self-aggrandizement.

Neither woman responded with any self-praise, but instead with great humility, insisting their actions were ordinary responses to a difficult situation. "My dad means everything to me," said Kornacki. "I'm having a hard time with this attention" (cited in Newcomb, 2012, online). When there is extreme non-narcissistic focus on the other, with a strong emotional connection, and no dilution of aim by self-aggrandizement or extraneous thoughts, it is possible that an individual may become an open vehicle for nonconsciously directed action.

Extraordinary Human Strength and the Philosophy of Yoga

When saving their fathers' lives, both Heffelmire and Kornacki were in a non-egotistical other-directed altered state generated by an intense focus on their fathers' welfare with no thought of themselves. This experience, which entailed lifting a multi-thousand-pound vehicle, appears to be congruent with certain aspects of advanced yoga practice. They are the attainment of *vibhuti* or extraordinary powers, such as strength (Eliade, 1969b). These abilities, which may arise in relationship with an object of extreme concentration (Patanjali, 2011), appeared to manifest in Heffelmire and Kornacki to help a father in peril.

An advanced yoga practitioner evidencing these powers would be in a state beyond trance. Yet in his treatise on the philosophy and consciousness of yoga, the *Yoga Sutra* (2011), Patanjali says *vibhuti* are not exclusive to yoga practice but may appear spontaneously in other situations. He believes the appearance of extraordinary powers, such as physical strength, traveling through space, or shrinking "to the size of an atom" (p. 56), arise when there is the formless integration of a person with an object. For Heffelmire and Kornacki, the concentrated one-pointed absorption with an object was their extreme focus on a father in need.

Patanjali writes (p. 105), "Concentration, absorption, and integration regarding a single object compose the perfect discipline of consciousness." Yet the combination of these advanced yoga practices which form samyama comes with an inherent danger (Eliade, 1975). There is a risk that the vibhuti, also known as siddhi, may become a source of pride and an end in themselves, obstructing spiritual advancement. There does not appear to be any suggestion of this in Heffelmire and Kornacki, both of whom showed great humility in deflecting any attention away from themselves and their accomplishments.

EHS: Heffelmire and a Buddhist Mantra, *Om Mani Padme Hum*

When Heffelmire was asked in a television interview (Daily Telegraph, 2021), where she found the physical and emotional strength to save her father, she said that she chanted *Om Mani Padme Hum* during the rescue, because her father told her to recite it in times of stress. It is a mantra associated with a calming response and altered states of consciousness (Pereira, 2016). Yet because Heffelmire is a great fan of the Seattle Seahawks football team, she changed it to *Om Mani Padme Russel* for their quarterback Russel Wilson. Heffelmire explained that "he's so calm in every situation, so I just channeled that." Wilson tweeted a commendation in response (cited in Seahawks.com, 2016), calling Heffelmire "a legend, a hero."

The words that Heffelmire chanted had great relevance to her situation. *Om Mani Padme Hum*, often translated as *Hail the Jewel in the Lotus*, is a Tibetan Buddhist mantra to invoke the bodhisattva Avalokiteshvara (Blofeld, 1970, 1978; Pereira, 2016). Embodying the active aspect of compassion, the deity is frequently sought by those in distress. Avalokiteshvara, who was born fully formed from a ray of light emanating from the right eye of Amitabha Buddha, is masculine in Tibet, but feminine in eastern Asia. Widely revered, her Sanskrit name translated into Chinese is Kwan Shih Yin, meaning *She-Who-Hearkens-to-the-Cries-of-the-World* (cited in Blofeld, 1978, p. 17), and more often as Kwan Yin, *Hearer-of-Cries*.

Extraordinary Human Strength: An Open Mind and the Energy of Inspiration

Another possible way to understand the phenomenon of extraordinary human strength is to note that its purposeful actions seem to be devoid of extraneous thoughts and appear to occur with an open mind. We usually associate openness of mind with meditation (Suzuki, 1973; Hanh, 1974), but any state, moving or still, that achieves non-distracted availability may be considered an open mind. Possibly, this opening may allow the rescuer to become an unimpeded vehicle, a conduit for energy. Siegel (2009) suggests this energy may arise from profound inspiration generated by a great purpose and occurring in trance. He cites the source for this concept as the *Yoga Sutras* of Patanjali and says (p. 88), "True inspiration overrides all fears. When you are inspired, you enter a trance state and can accomplish things that you may never have felt capable of doing."

For Heffelmire and Kornacki, an experience of extreme emotion may have generated a profound inspiration to rescue. When creative people become vehicles for their inspiration it energizes them. Extraordinary human strength, with its creative problem-solving, also appears to be an inspired state. Yet here the physical energy is enormous and seems to arise in response to a change of consciousness occurring during the rescue effort. As evidenced by Heffelmire and Kornacki, the emotion of great panic at the thought of losing someone, combined with selfless love and devotion vastly overrides any thoughts of the self or personal welfare. This emotionally energized selfless response may shift the consciousness of the rescuer to an altered state where they have access to or become conduits for an enormous source of energy.

Extraordinary Human Strength and the Model of a Singularity

The energy in extraordinary human strength may possibly arise through dynamics like those of a singularity. A singularity is a point in space-time, such as the center in a black hole, where matter can be so infinitely concentrated that the ordinary laws of physics no longer apply. When a massive star, at least five times the size of our sun, reaches the end of its life and collapses its matter intensely, it may become a black hole (NASA, 2017). Progressing from star to black hole entails a fundamental change in its state of being. Transforming from something that is governed by the rules of ordinary space-time to something that is not, it becomes an ontological mutation in the linearity of existence.

While ontological mutations in linear existence are a known phenomenon in astrophysics, it is possible that they may also occur during times of extremely concentrated consciousness, such as the one-pointed focus in a lifesaving creative trance. A black hole exists for an extended amount of time, and extraordinary human strength is a short-term event, yet they both contain phenomena that appear to be beyond the physics of our space-time. Not only did both women lift a multi-thousand-pound vehicle and pull a grown man out from under it, but their experience of its weight was not ordinary. Heffelmire said the truck was as light as a piece of paper and Kornacki compared lifting the vehicle to lifting one leg of a table and balancing it on the other three.

Both women were in ordinary consciousness before discovering a father in peril and returned to daily awareness after the event. Yet during the extreme state of a lifesaving creative trance, it appears as if their highly focused consciousness temporarily progressed to a type of psychological singularity where the ordinary laws of physics were suspended. This suggests that in certain extreme altered states, consciousness may change its state of being, and analogous to the progression of massive stars, become an ontological mutation in the linearity of existence. If there is a dynamic such as a psychological singularity that may provide access to the power of extraordinary human strength, the following discussion investigates possible sources that might fuel its energy.

Aspects of EHS and the Ubiquitous Energy Field

The personal power evidenced in extraordinary human strength appears to be vastly beyond any normal parameters and yet it is also time limited. Marie "Bootsy" Payton easily threw the riding lawnmower off her trapped granddaughter but could not even move the machine later when there was no child to save. Tom Boyle, Jr., who lifted a Camaro to save a cyclist caught beneath it, said later in an interview that he could no longer lift the car. These incidents suggest that the source of energy may not reside within the person but possibly have an external origin that was accessible when needed to save a life.

The external energy source for these extreme feats of strength would have to be ubiquitous, enormous, and possibly also time limited. Ubiquitous because the incidents occur in different people, places, and times, enormous because of the prodigious capabilities involved, and time limited or borrowed because it appears to only last long enough to save a life. In contemporary Western thought, these qualities may suggest a quantum source of power, perhaps deriving from the energy inherent in the pervasive quantum field.

Aspects of this field are called the void, dark energy, vacuum energy, or zero-point energy. It is universally prevalent, potentially huge, and characterized by multiple short-term energy interactions. The energy field exists because empty space is not empty but filled with constant activity. What is termed a void or dark energy is instead a plenipotential ground of seething movement. Generating and absorbing particles, it is an endless dance of creation, annihilation, and recreation.

Theories of Exterior and Interior Quantum Processes

There may be a possible connection between quantum fields, such as zero-point energy fields, and hypothesized quantum processes in the brain. One of the current theories of quantum brain processes is the Penrose-Hameroff formulation of orchestrated objective reduction (Hameroff & Penrose, 1996; Penrose & Hameroff, 2011). Known as Orch OR, it postulates that consciousness is central to the physical universe, has always been in the universe, and plays an intrinsic role in the functioning of laws in the universe. Penrose and Hameroff believe consciousness originates from objective reduction, a quantum process orchestrated by assemblies of microtubules, which are cellular structures found inside brain neurons. They suggest the microtubules, which are protein polymers, function as a biomolecular computer regulating neuronal activity.

Fisher (2015) hypothesizes quantum processing occurs in the brain through the nuclear spins of phosphorus, with the phosphate ion acting as a neural qubit-transporter. He suggests that the "Posner molecule," $Ca_9(PO_4)_6$, can protect the phosphate ion in the warm wet brain environment and believes that the entanglement of multiple Posner molecules may activate neural quantum processing.

Meijer and Geesink (2017) theorize that the brain is a hyper-dimensional structure with a field-receptive, extra-corporal, nonmaterial mental workspace. They postulate that this workspace interacts with zero-point energy, dark energy, and other energy fields, and that these interactions become a foundation for consciousness. In their theory, the brain is rooted in a holographic field and its mental workspace, which is also holographic, receives information through a "brain event horizon" (p. 41). Relevant to the observation that extraordinary human strength appears to arise from a nonconscious source is Meijer and Geesink's (2017, p. 42) belief that "the central nervous system is embedded in a much wider context in which it also receives (quantum) wave information, partly unrelated to the known senses." They note that quantum information is a type of energy and postulate that living systems are organized energy information fields.

Extraordinary Human Strength and Cultural Correlates to the Energy Field

The concept that humans are energy fields inhabiting a larger energy-filled universe is archaic and cross-cultural. The plenipotential void has been a subject of Western culture since the ancient Greek civilization. In his Atomist Doctrine, the philosopher Democritus (b. 460 BCE) believed that the great void was not empty but filled with an infinite number of constantly moving indestructible atoms colliding, repelling, and combining with each other (Berryman, 2016). There is also the concept of a plenipotential void in contemporary physics, which has similarities to the idea of a universal field in Eastern philosophy (Capra, 1975).

As the Song dynasty scholar Chang Tsai (Zhang Zai, 1020–1077) states, "When one knows that the great void is full of chi, one realizes that there is no such thing as nothingness" (cited in Capra, 1975, p. 223). In Eastern philosophy, everything in the universe is made of ch'i and enlivened by it, making universal ch'i energies available to human beings. The open-minded yet focused trance states of Heffelmire and Kornacki may have greatly enhanced the flow of ch'i, both into them and through them. As the Neo-Confucian scholar Lu Chiu-yuan (Lù Jiǔyuān, 1139–1192) believes, "The universe is my mind and my mind is the universe" (cited in Tang Chün-I, 1956, p. 115).

In classical Indian philosophy and the Ayurvedic tradition there is also a connection between the mind and the universe, where the mind is a field able to receive great strength and energy (Shamasundar, 2008). Yet most people do not experience their field-like mind, because it is hidden by a preoccupation with the material concerns of daily life. Immersion in the fleeting distractions of materiality can obscure the subtleness and sensitivity necessary for extraordinary events. In their altered states, Heffelmire and Kornacki did not think of daily life or themselves, but only concentrated on rescuing a father. For the Ayurvedic and classical Indian traditions, this would suggest a focused open mind, capable of achieving and exercising the enormous capacities that are always available to us. When these strengths manifest during the altered states of a creative trance, we realize that we have the possibilities to be far more than we are or even imagined we could be.

References

Aaron, P. G., Phillips, S. & Larsen, S. (1988). Specific reading disability in historically famous persons. *Journal of Learning Disabilities*, 21(9), 253–538.

Abell, A. M. (1994). *Talks with great composers.* New York: Carol (original work published 1955).

Abraham, A. (2018). *The neuroscience of creativity.* Cambridge: Cambridge University Press.

Abraham, F. D. (2016). *Microcosm of the psyche.* Paper presented at the International Center for the Study of Archetypal Patterns, Assisi Institute.

Abraham, F. D., Abraham, R. H. & Shaw, C. (1989). *A visual introduction to dynamical systems theory for psychology.* Santa Cruz: Aerial Press.

Ackerman, D. (1990). *A natural history of the senses.* New York: Random House.

Acquadro, M. A. S., Congedo, M. & De Riddeer, D. (2016). Music performance as an experimental approach to hyperscanning studies. *Frontiers in Human Neuroscience*, 10, 242.

Adams, T. (2010). Sargy Mann: The blind painter of Peckham. *The Guardian* www.theguardian.com.

Aesop. (1969). The crow and the pitcher. In C. W. Eliot (ed.), *Folk-lore and fable: Aesop, Grim, Andersen.* New York: P. F. Collier, 32 (original work published 1909).

Alexander, M. E., Ackerman, M. Y. & Baxter, G. J. (2009). *An analysis of Dodge's escape fire on the 1949 Mann Gulch Fire in terms of a survival zone for wildland fighters.* Paper presented at the 10th Wildland Fire Safety Summit, International Association of Wildland Fire, Phoenix, Arizona.

Allen, M. P. (2017). *Transcendents: Spirit mediums in Burma and Thailand.* Durham: Daylight Books.

Allen, M. P. (2021). Voices from the collections: Photographer Mariette Pathy Allen in conversation with curator Makeda Best. *Harvard Museum.* https://harvardartmuseums.org.

Alter, A. (2020). He invented the Rubik's Cube. He's still learning from it. *The New York Times.* www.nytimes.com.

Amaducci, L., Grassi, E. & Boller, F. (2002). Maurice Ravel and right-hemisphere musical creativity: Influence of disease on his last musical works? *European Journal of Neurology*, 9(1), 75–82. x.

Amâncio, E. J. (2005). Dostoevsky and Stendhal's syndrome. *Arquivos Neuropsiquiatr*, 63(4), 1099–1103.

American Heart Association News Archive. (2014). Stories from the heart: Lifting a 3,500-pound car was only the start to saving her dad's life; knowing CPR made a difference, too. https://newsarchive.heart.org.

American Psychiatric Association (ed.). (2013). *DSM-5: Diagnostic and statistical manual of mental disorders*, 5th ed. Washington: American Psychiatric Association.

American Psychological Association (APA). (2020). APA dictionary of psychology. https://dictionary.apa.org.

Anderson, R. & Hanrahan, S. J. (2008). Dancing in pain: Pain appraisal and coping in dancers. *Journal of Dance Medicine & Science*, 12(1), 9–16.

Anderson-Maples, J. (2019). UAH welcomes Bob Lujano Paralympic medalist to campus. *University of Alabama in Huntsville News*. www.uah.edu/news.

Antl-Weiser, W. (2009). The time of the Willendorf figurines and new results of Palaeolithic research in Lower Austria. *Anthropologie*, 47(1/2), 131–141.

Appenzeller, T. (1998). Art: Evolution or revolution? *Science*, 282(5393), 1451–1454.

Archer, S. (2009). "I had a terror": Emily Dickinson's demon. *Southwest Review*, 94(2), 255–273.

Archive for Research in Archetypal Symbolism (ARAS). (2020). Egg. https://aras .org.

ArtsProfessional. (2020). Arts professionals recognised in New Year honours. www .artsprofessional.co.uk.

Austen, R. (2013). Celebrating Balanchine: Getting to know Mr. B. *Oregon Ballet Theatre*. www.obt.org

Automaticity. (2007). In *APA dictionary of psychology*. https://dictionary.apa.org.

AXIS Dance. (2020). AXIS dance company. www.axisdance.org.

Bachrach, A., Fontbonne, Y., Joufflineau, C. & Ulloa, J. L. (2015). Audience entrainment during live contemporary dance performance: Physiological and cognitive measures. *Frontiers in Human Neuroscience*, 9, 179.

Bagby, R. M., Costa, P. T., Widiger, T. A., Ryder, A. G. & Marshall, M. (2005). DSM-IV personality disorders and the five-factor model of personality: A multi-method examination of domain- and facet-level predictions. *European Journal of Personality*, 19, 307–324.

Baird, A. & Thompson, W. F. (2019). When music compensates language: A case study of severe aphasia in dementia and the use of music by a spousal caregiver. *Aphasiology*, 33(4), 449–465.

Bak, P. (1996). *How nature works: The science of self-organized criticality*. New York: Copernicus.

Bak, P., Tang, C. & Wiesenfeld, K. (1988). Self-organized criticality. *Physical Review. A*, 38, 364–374.

Baldwin, J. (1962). The creative process. In J. F. Kennedy (ed.), *Creative America*. New York: Ridge Press, 16–21.

Balme, J. & Morse, K. (2006). Shell beads and social behaviour in Pleistocene Australia. *Antiquity*, 80, 799–811.

Balter, M. (2015). World's oldest stone tools discovered in Kenya. *Science*.

Bambach, C. C. (2003a). Introduction to Leonardo and his drawings. In C. C. Bambach (ed.), *Leonardo da Vinci: Master draftsman*, The Metropolitan Museum of Art. New Haven: Yale University Press, 3–30.

Bambach, C. C. (2003b). Leonardo, left-handed draftsman and writer. In C. C. Bambach (ed.), *Leonardo da Vinci: Master draftsman*, The Metropolitan Museum of Art. New Haven: Yale University Press, 31–57.

Bandura, A. (1997). *Self-efficacy: The exercise of control*. New York: W. H. Freeman.

Banissy, M. J. (2013). Synaesthesia, mirror neurons, and mirror-touch. In J. Simner & E. M. Hubbard (eds.), *The Oxford handbook of synesthesia*. Oxford: Oxford University Press, 585–603.

Bannister, R. (2018). *The four minute mile*. Guilford: Lyons Press (original work published 1955)

Barber, M. (2020). Taka Suzuki keen to pull right "strings" for home glory. *Paralympic News*. World Para Swimming, Paralympic Organization. www .paralympic.org.

Bargh, J. A. (2005). Bypassing the will: Toward demystifying the nonconscious control of social behavior. In R. R. Hassin, J. S. Uleman & J. A. Bargh (eds.), *The new unconscious*. New York: Oxford University Press, 37–58.

Bargh, J. A. & Chartrand, T. L. (1999). The unbearable automaticity of being. *American Psychologist*, 54(7), 462–479.

Bargh, J. A. & Williams, E. L. (2006). The automaticity of social life. *Current Directions in Psychological Science*, 15(1), 1–4.

Barrett, D. (1993). The "committee of sleep": A study of dream incubation for problem solving. *Journal of the Association for the Study of Dreams*, 2(3), 115–123.

Barrett, D. (2010). *The committee of sleep*. Oneiroi Press.

Barriquand, L., Bigot, J.-Y., Audra, P. et al. (2021). Caves and bats: Morphological impacts and archaeological implications. The Azé Prehistoric Cave (Saône-et-Loire, France). *Geomorphology*, 388, 107785.

Barron, F. (1969). *Creative person and creative process*. New York: Holt, Rinehart, and Winston.

Barron, F., Montuori, A. & Barron, A. (1997). *Creators on creating*. New York: Tarcher/Penguin.

Baruss, I. (2003). *Alterations of consciousness: An empirical analysis for social scientists*. Washington: American Psychological Association.

Baruss, I. & Mossbridge, J. (2017). *Transcendent mind: Rethinking the science of consciousness*. Washington: American Psychological Association.

Bar-Yosef Mayer, D. E., Bernard Vandermeersch, B. & Bar-Yosef, O. (2009). Shells and ochre in Middle Paleolithic Qafzeh Cave, Israel: indications for modern behavior. *Journal of Human Evolution*, 56(3), 307–314.

Baseball Hall of Fame. (n.d.). Lou Brock. https://baseballhall.org.

Basso, J. C., Satyal, M. K. & Rugh, R. (2021). Dance on the brain: Enhancing intra- and inter-brain synchrony. *Frontiers in Human Neuroscience*, 14, 584312.

Battalı, C., Occelli, V., Bertonati, G., Falagiarda, F. & Collignon, O. (2020). General enhancement of spatial hearing in congenitally blind people. *Psychological Science*, 31(9), 1129–1139.

Bayley, H. (1988). *The lost language of symbolism*. Secaucus: Citadel Press.

Bayley, J. (1999). *Elegy for Iris*. London: Picador.

Bearden, R. (1976). *Horace Pippin*. Essay in the exhibition catalog *Horace Pippin*. Washington: The Phillips Collection.

Beaton, A. (2004). *Dyslexia, reading and the brain: A sourcebook of psychological and biological research*. Hove: Psychology Press.

Beaty, R. E., Benedek, M., Wilkins, R. W. et al. (2014). Creativity and the default network: A functional connectivity analysis. *Neuropsychologia*, 64, 29–98.

Beaty, R. E., Kaufman, S. B., Benedek, M. et al. (2016). Personality and complex brain networks: The role of openness to experience in default network efficiency. *Human Brain Mapping*, 37, 773–779.

Beauregard, M. & O'Leary, D. (2007). *The spiritual brain: A neuroscientist's case for the existence of the soul*. New York: HarperOne.

Beauregard, M. & Paquette, V. (2006). Neural correlates of a mystical experience in Carmelite nuns. *Neuroscience Letters*, 405(3), 186–190.

Beauregard, M., Trent, N. L. & Schwartz, G. E. (2018). Toward a postmaterialist psychology: Theory, research, and applications. *New Ideas in Psychology*, 50, 21–33.

Bednarik, R. G. (1998). The "Australopithecine" cobble from Makapansgat, South Africa. *The South African Archaeological Bulletin*, 53(167), 4.

Bednarik, R. G. (2003). A figurine from the African Acheulian. *Current Anthropology*, 44(3), 405–413.

Bednarik, R. G. (2010). Estimating the age of cupules. In R. Q. Lewis & R. G. Bednarik (eds.), *Mysterious cup marks: Proceedings of the First International Cupule Conference*, BAR International Series 2073. Oxford: Archaeopress, 5–12.

Beethoven, L. van. (2008). *Beethoven's letters*. L. Wallace (trans.). Kindle ed. Oxford: Archaeopress.

Beilock, S. L., Carr, T. H., MacMahon, C. & Starkes, J. L. (2002). When paying attention becomes counterproductive: Impact of divided versus skill-focused attention on novice and experienced performance of sensorimotor skills. *Journal of Experimental Psychology: Applied*, 8, 6–16.

Berman, J. (Spring/Summer 2000). Red salmon and red cedar bark: Another look at the nineteenth-century Kwakwaka'wakw winter ceremonial. *BC Studies*, 125 (6), 53–99.

Berryman, S. (Winter 2016). Democritus. In E. N. Zalta (ed.), *The Stanford Encyclopedia of Philosophy*. https://plato.stanford.edu.

Bhattacharya, K. & Neela, C. N. (2006). Da Vinci's code for surgeons. *Indian Journal of Surgery*, 68(5), 284–285.

Bierer, L. M., Hof, P. R., Purohit, D. P. et al. (1995). Neocortical neurofibrillary tangles correlate with dementia severity in Alzheimer's disease. *Archives of Neurology*, 52(1), 81–88.

Binyon, L. (1969). *Painting in the Far East*. New York: Dover (original work published 1934).

Bird, C. D. & Emery, N. J. (2009). Insightful problem solving and creative tool modification by captive nontool-using rooks. *Proceedings of the National Academy of Sciences*, 106(25), 10370–10375. .

Black, J. (1993). Reflections on the analytical pharmacology of histamine h2-receptor antagonists. *Gastroenterology*, 105, 963–998.

Blake, W. (1820). *For the sexes: The gates of paradise*. London: Illuminated manuscript published by William Blake (original work published 1793, plates added 1820).

Blakey, D. N. (2016). *Blind Willie Johnson – the biography: Revelation the man the words the music*. Amazon Kindle ed. (original work published 2007).

Blofeld, J. (1970). *The tantric mysticism of Tibet*. New York: E. P. Dutton.

Blofeld, J. (1978). *Bodhisattva of compassion: The mystical tradition of Kwan Yin*. Boston: Shambhala.

Boas, F. (1955). *Primitive art*. New York: Dover (original work published 1927).

Bolhuis, J. J., Tattersall, I., Chomsky, N. & Berwick, R. C. (2014). How could language have evolved? *PLoS Biol*, 12(8), e1001934.

Bonta, M., Gosford, R., Eussen, D. et al. (2017). Intentional fire-spreading by fire hawk raptors in northern Australia. *Journal of Ethnobiology*, 37(4), 700–718.

Boso, M., Enzo, E., Minazzi, V., Abbamonte, M. & Politi, P. (2007).Effect of long-term interactive music therapy on behavior profile and musical skills in young adults with severe autism. *The Journal of Alternative and Complementary Medicine*, 13(7), 709–712.

Bourne, E. J. (2020). *The anxiety and phobia workbook*, 7th ed. Oakland: New Harbinger.

Bowie, H. P. (1952). *On the laws of Japanese painting*. New York: Dover (original work published 1911).

Bowman, F. L. & Culotta, V. (2010). Self-assessment tool. *The International Dyslexia Association*. www.interdys.org.

Brahmavamso, A. (2005). *The Jhanas*. Penang: Inward Path.

Briggs, J. & Peat, F. D. (1989). *Turbulent mirror*. New York: Harper & Row.

British Council. (2020). Europe beyond access. *Disability Arts International*. www .disabilityartsinternational.org.

Brown, E. (1989). *Albert Pinkham Ryder*. Washington: The Smithsonian Institution Press.

Brown, T. E. (2005). *Attention deficit disorder: The unfocused mind in children and adults*. New Haven: Yale University Press, Kindle ed.

Buehler, M. J. (2020). Nanomechanical sonification of the 2019-nCoV coronavirus spike protein through a materiomusical approach. *Cornell University, arXiv*. https://arxiv.org.

Burgoon, J. K. & White, C. E. (2013). Researching nonverbal message production: A view from interaction adaptation theory. In J. O. Greene (ed.), *Message production: Advances in communication theory*. New York: Routledge Communication Series, Kindle ed., 279–312.

Burns, C. (ed.). (2008). *Off the page: Writers talk about beginnings, endings, and everything in between*. New York: W. W. Norton.

Burrage, C., Copeland, E. J. & Hinds, E. A. (2015). Probing dark energy with atom interferometry. *Journal of Cosmology and Astroparticle Physics*, 3 (42), 1–20.

Burroughs, E. R. (2014). *The mad king: "Imagination is but another name for super intelligence."* Horse's Mouth Books (original work published 1914).

Butter, C. M., Trobe, J. D., Foster, N. L. & Berent, S. (1996). Visual-spatial deficits explain visual symptoms in Alzheimer's disease. *American Journal of Ophthalmology*, 122(1), 97–105.

Cacioppo, J. T., Norris, C. J., Decety, J., Monteleone, G. & Nusbaum, H. (2009). In the eye of the beholder: Individual differences in perceived social isolation predict regional brain activation to social stimuli. *Journal of Cognitive Neuroscience*, 21(1), 83–92.

Capra, F. (1975). *The tao of physics*. Berkeley: Shambhala.

Cardarelli, S. & Fenelli, L. (2017). *Saints, miracles, and the image: Healing saints and miraculous images in the Renaissance*. Turnhout: Brepols.

Cardeña, E. (1997). The etiologies of dissociation. In S. Krippner & S. M. Powers (eds.), *Broken images, broken selves: Dissociative narratives in clinical practice*. Washington: Brunner/Mazel, 61–87.

Cardeña, E., Iribas, A. E. & Reijman, S. (2012). Art and psi. *Journal of Parapsychology*, 76, 3–25.

Caruana, W. (1993). *Aboriginal art*. New York: Thames and Hudson.

Cavallera, G. M., Giudici, S. & Tommasi, L. (2012). Shadows and darkness in the brain of a genius: Aspects of the neuropsychological literature about the final illness of Maurice Ravel (1875–1937). *Medical Science Monitor*, 18(10), MH1–MH8.

Centers for Disease Control and prevention (CDC). (2020). U.S. public health service syphilis study at Tuskegee: The Tuskegee timeline. www.cdc.gov.

Champigneulle, B. (1967). *Rodin*. New York: Oxford University Press, 14.

Chang, C.-y. (1970). *Creativity and taoism: A study of Chinese philosophy, art, and poetry*. New York: Harper & Row.

Cheney, M. (1981). *Tesla: Man out of time*. New York: Barnes & Noble Books.

Chevalier, J. & Gheerbrant, A. (eds.). (1996). *The Penguin dictionary of symbols*. J. Buchannan-Brown (trans.). London: Penguin Books.

Christie, A. (2010). *Agatha Christie: An autobiography*. New York: HarperCollins e-books (original work published 1977).

Christie, A. (2020). About Agatha Christie. *The home of Agatha Christie*. www.agathachristie.com.

Chun, C. A. & Hupe, J.-M. (2016). Are synesthetes exceptional beyond their synesthetic associations? A systematic comparison of creativity, personality, cognition, and mental imagery in synesthetes and controls. *British Journal of Psychology*, 107, 397–418.

Cirlot, J. E. (1971). *A dictionary of symbols*. J. Sage (trans.). New York: Philosophical Library.

Clare, Y. (2017). Stanislavsky's system as an enactive guide to embodied cognition? *Connection Science*, 29(1), 43–63.

Claridge, L. (2001). *Norman Rockwell: A life*. New York: Random House.

Clark, J. (2019). How can adrenaline help you lift a 3,500-pound car? *Howstuffworks* https://entertainment.howstuffworks.com.

Clayton, N. S., Bussey, T. J. & Dickinson, A. (2003). Can animals recall the past and plan for the future? *Nature Reviews Neuroscience*, 4, 685–691.

Clift, S. & Morrison, I. (2011). Group singing fosters mental health and wellbeing: findings from the East Kent "singing for health" network project. *Mental Health and Social Inclusion*, 15(2), 88–97.

Clottes, J. (2016). *What is Paleolithic art? Cave paintings and the dawn of human creativity*. O. Y. Martin & R. D. Martin (trans.). Chicago: University of Chicago Press.

Clottes, J. & Lewis-Williams, D. (1998). *The shamans of prehistory: Trance and magic in the painted caves*. S. Hawkes (trans.). New York: Harry N. Abrams.

CNN Wire Staff. (2012). Woman lifts car, saves her father. www.cnn.com.

Cognitive Neuroscience. (2007). In *APA dictionary of psychology*. https://dictionary.apa.org.

Cognitive Unconscious. (2007). In *APA dictionary of psychology*. https://dictionary.apa.org.

Cohen, D. & Schmidt, J. P. (1979). Ambiversion: Characteristics of midrange responders on the introversion-extraversion continuum. *Journal of Personality Assessment*, 43(5), 514–516.

Coleridge, S. T. (1985). Prefatory note to Kublai Khan. In B. Ghiselin (ed.), *The creative process*. Berkeley: University of California Press, 83–84 (original work published 1946).

Colman, E. (1998). Obesity in the Paleolithic era? The Venus of Willendorf. *Endocrine Practice*, 4(1), 58–59.

Combs, A. & Krippner, S. (2003). Process, structure, and form: An evolutionary transpersonal psychology of consciousness. *International Journal of Transpersonal Studies*, 22(1), 47–60.

Combs, A. & Krippner, S. (2007). Structures of consciousness and creativity: Opening the doors of perception. In R. Richards (ed.), *Everyday creativity and new vies of human nature: Psychological, social, and spiritual perspectives*. Washington: American Psychological Association, 131–149.

Combs, A. L. (2002). *The radiance of being: Understanding the grand integral vision; Living the integral life*. St. Paul: Paragon House.

Congreve, W. (2017). *The mourning bride: Tragic drama*. Scotts Valley: CreateSpace Independent (original work published 1697).

Consciousness. (2007). In *APA dictionary of psychology*. https://dictionary.apa.org.

Cooke, J. F. (1999). *Great Pianists on piano playing: Godowsky, Hofmann, Lhevinne, Paderewski and 24 other legendary performers*. New York: Dover Books on Music (original work published 1917).

Corballis, M. (2018). Laterality and creativity: A false trail? In R. E. Jung & O. Vartanian (eds.), *The Cambridge handbook of the neuroscience of creativity*. Cambridge: Cambridge University Press, 50–57.

Corley, C. (2010). Creative expression and resilience among Holocaust survivors. *Journal of Human Behavior in the Social Environment*, 20, 542–552.

Cortese, S., Kelly, C., Chabernaud, C. et al. (2012). Toward systems neuroscience of ADHD: A meta-analysis of 55 fMRI studies. *The American Journal of Psychiatry*. 169(10), 1038–1055.

Cramond, B. (1994). Attention deficit hyperactivity disorder and creativity – What is the connection? *The Journal of Creative Behavior*, 28(3), 193–210.

Cropley, D. H., Kaufman, J. C. & Cropley, A. J. (2008). Malevolent creativity: A functional model of creativity in terrorism and crime. *Creativity Research Journal*, 20(2), 105–115.

Crowe, T. & Wells, F. (2004). Leonardo da Vinci as a paradigm for modern clinical research. *The Journal of Thoracic and Cardiovascular Surgery*, 127(4), 929–994.

Crutch, S. J., Isaacs, R. & Rossor, M. J. (2001). Some workmen can blame their tools: Artistic change in an individual with Alzheimer's disease. *The Lancet*, 357, 2129–2133.

Csikszentmihalyi, M. (1990). *Flow: The psychology of optimal experience*. New York: Harper & Row.

Csikszentmihalyi, M. (1996). *Creativity: Flow and the psychology of discovery and invention*. New York: HarperCollins.

Cullon, D. (2013). A view from the watchman's pole: Salmon, animism and the Kwakwaka'wakw summer ceremonial. *BC Studies*, [s. l.], (177), 9–37.

Currey, M. (2014). *Daily rituals: How artists work*. New York: Knopf.

Currey, M. (2019). *Daily rituals: Women at work*. New York: Knopf.

Curtin, A. (2015). "O body swayed to music": The allure of Jacqueline du Pré as spectacle and drama. *Studies in Musical Theatre*, 9(2), 143–159.

Cytowic, R. E. (2002). *Synesthesia: A union of the senses*. Cambridge: MIT Press.

Cytowic, R. E. (2018). *Synesthesia*. Cambridge: MIT Press.

Czeszumski, A., Eustergerling, S., Lang, A. et al. (2020). Hyperscanning: A valid method to study neural inter-brain underpinnings of social interaction. *Frontiers in Human Neuroscience*, 14, 39.

Daily Telegraph. (2021). Teen "superwoman" lifts pickup truck to save dad from fire. www.dailytelegraph.com.au/news (original work published 2016).

Dance for PD. (2020). Dance for PD: A program of the Mark Morris Dance Group. https://danceforparkinsons.org.

Dart, R. A. (1974). The waterworn Australopithecine pebble of many faces from Makapansgat. *South African Journal of Science*, 70, 167–169

David, A. R. (2009). Performing for the gods? Dance and embodied ritual in British Hindu temples. *South Asian Popular Culture*, 7(3), 217–231.

David-Neel, A. (1971). *Magic and mystery in Tibet*. The Bodley Head (trans.). Baltimore: Penguin Books (original work published 1929).

David-Neel, A. (1970). *Initiations and initiates in Tibet*. F. Rothwell (trans.). Berkeley: Shambhala (original work published 1930).

Davidson, I. J. (Autumn 2017). The ambivert: A failed attempt at a normal personality. *Journal of the History of the Behavioral Sciences*, 53(4), 313–331.

Davidson, R. J. & Lutz, A. (2008). Buddha's brain: Neuroplasticity and meditation. *IEEE Signal Processing Magazine*, 25(1), 174–176.

Davis, E., Loiacono, R. & Summers, R. J. (2008). The rush to adrenaline: Drugs in sport acting on the b-adrenergic system. *British Journal of Pharmacology*, 154, 584–597.

Davis, J. (2016). The primordial mandalas of East and West: Jungian and Tibetan Buddhist approaches to healing and transformation. *NeuroQuantology: An Interdisciplinary Journal of Neuroscience and Quantum Physics*, 14(2), 242–254.

de Arcangelis, L., Perrone-Capano, C. & Herrmann, H. J. (2006). Self-organized criticality model for brain plasticity. *Physical Review Letters*, 96, 028107.

De Bono, E. (1990). *Lateral thinking: A textbook of creativity*. London: Penguin Books (original work published 1970).

Decker, E. (2019). Group singing provides a good refrain for the brain. *International Arts + Mind Lab (IAM Lab), Johns Hopkins Medicine*. www.artsandmindlab.org.

Decker, E. (2020). The arts can liberate us from loneliness. *International Arts + Mind Lab (IAM Lab), Johns Hopkins Medicine*. www.artsandmindlab.org.

Defense mechanism. (2007). In *APA dictionary of psychology*. https://dictionary.apa.org.

DeGeneres, E. (2016). Charlotte Heffelmire visits Ellen. *The Ellen DeGeneres Show, NBC Washington, NBC4*. https://hu-hu.facebook.com/nbcwashington/videos.

Dehaene, S. (2014). *Consciousness and the brain: Deciphering how the brain codes our thoughts*. New York: Penguin Books.

De Heinzelin, J., Desmond, J. C., White, T. et al. (1999). Environment and behavior of 2.5-million-year-old Bouri Hominids. *Science*, 284(5414), 625–629.

Demertzi, A., Tagliazucchi, E., Dehaene, S. et al. (2019) Human consciousness is supported by dynamic complex patterns of brain signal coordination. *Science Advances*, Published online.

Deniz, F., Nunez-Elizalde, A. O., Huth, A. G. & Gallant, J. L. (2019). The representation of semantic information across human cerebral cortex during listening versus reading is invariant to stimulus modality. *Journal of Neuroscience*, 39(39), 7722–7736. .

De Pascalis, V., Paolo, S. & Arianna Vecchio, A. (2021). Influences of hypnotic suggestibility, contextual factors, and EEG alpha on placebo analgesia. *American Journal of Clinical Hypnosis*, 63(4), 302–328.

De Pascalis, V., Scacchia, P. & Vecchio, A. (2021). Influences of hypnotic suggestibility, contextual factors, and EEG alpha on placebo analgesia. *American Journal of Clinical Hypnosis*, 63(4), 302–328.

d'Errico, F., Henshilwood, C., Lawson, G. et al. (2003). Archaeological evidence for the emergence of language, symbolism, and music – An alternative multi-disciplinary perspective. *Journal of World Prehistory*, 17(1), 2–67.

d'Errico, F., Henshilwood, C. & Nilssen, P. (2001). An engraved bone fragment from c. 70,000-year-old Middle Stone Age levels at Blombos Cave, South Africa: Implications for the origin of symbolism and language. *Antiquity*, 75 (288), 309–318.

d'Errico, F. & Nowell, A. (2000). A new look at the Berekhat Ram figurine: Implications for the origins of symbolism. *Cambridge Archaeological Journal*, 10, 123–167.

de Salas, X. (1981). *Goya*. A. Mondadori (trans.). New York: Mayflower Books.

Descargues, P. (1979). *Goya*. New York: Crescent Books.

De Vico Fallani, F., Nicosia, V., Sinatra, R. et al. (2010). Defecting or not defecting: How to "read" human behavior during cooperative games by EEG measurements. *PLoS ONE*, 5(12), e14187.

de Villiers, D., van Rooyen, F. C., Comm, M. et al. (2013). Wheelchair dancing and self-esteem in adolescents with physical disabilities. *South African Journal of Occupational Therapy*, 43(2), 23–27.

De Vries, A. (1984). *Dictionary of symbols and imagery*. Amsterdam: North-Holland.

Dewhurst, S., Nelson, N., Dougall, P. K. & Bampouras, T. (2014). Scottish country dance: Benefits to functional ability in older women. *Journal of Aging & Physical Activity*, 22(1), 146–153.

Di Biase, F. (2009). A holoinformational model of consciousness. *Quantum Biosystems*, 3, 207–220.

DiCarlo, J. J., Zoccolan, D. & Rust, N. C. (2012). How does the brain solve visual object recognition? *Neuron*, 73(3), 415–434.

Dickens, C. (1859). *David Copperfield*. Classic Books, Kindle ed.

Dickinson, E. (2015). *The complete poems of Emily Dickinson*. Radford: SMK Books, Kindle ed.

Dietrich, A. (2004). The cognitive neuroscience of creativity. *Psychonomic Bulletin & Review*, 11(6), 1011–1026.

Dissanayake, E. (1988). *What is art for?* Seattle: University of Washington Press.

Dissanayake, E. (1992). *Homo aestheticus: Where art comes from and why*. Seattle: University of Washington Press.

Dissociation. (2007). In *APA dictionary of psychology*. https://dictionary.apa.org.

Dissociative Trance Disorder. (2007). In *APA dictionary of psychology*. https://dictionary.apa.org.

Dixson, A. F. & Dixson, B. J. (2011). Venus figurines of the European Paleolithic: Symbols of fertility or attractiveness? *Journal of Anthropology*, 2011 (Article ID 569120), 11 pages.

Doctorow, E. L. (1988). Interview. In G. Plimpton (ed.), *Writers at work: The Paris review interviews, Eighth series*. New York: Penguin Books, 301–321.

Donald, M. (1991). *Origins of the modern mind: Three stages in the evolution of culture and cognition*. Cambridge: Harvard University Press.

Donald, M. (1995). The neurobiology of human consciousness: An evolutionary approach. *Neuropsychologia*, 33(9), 1087–1102.

Donald, M. (2006). Art and cognitive evolution. In M. Turner (ed.), *The artful mind: Cognitive science and the riddle of human creativity*. Oxford: Oxford University Press, 3–20.

Dossey, L. (1993). *Healing words: The power of prayer and the practice of medicine*. San Francisco: HarperSanFrancisco.

Dovern, A., Fink, G. R., Fromme, C. B. et al. (2012). Intrinsic network connectivity reflects consistency of synesthetic experiences. *The Journal of Neuroscience*, 32(22), 7614–7621.

Drob, S. L. (2000). The doctrine of Coincidentia Oppositorum in Jewish mysticism. *Kabbalah and Post Modernism*. www.newkabbalah.com.

Duchamp, M. (1973). The creative act. In M. Sanouillet & E. Peterson, *Salt seller: The writings of Marcel Duchamp*. New York: Oxford University Press, 138–140.

Duncan, I. (1997). Isadora Duncan: The mother cry of creation. In F. Barron, A. Montuori & A. Barron (eds.), *Creators on creating*. New York: Tarcher/Penguin, 207–208.

Dunkerton, J. (2011). Leonardo in Verrocchio's workshop: Re-examining the technical evidence. *National Gallery Technical Bulletin: Leonardo da Vinci: Pupil, Painter and Master*, 32, 4–31.

Durkheim, É. (1915). *The elementary forms of the religious life*. J. Swain (trans.). London: George Allen & Unwin, Kindle ed., 219

Dutton, D. (2010). The uses of fiction. In B. Boyd, J. Carroll & J. Gottshall (eds.), *Evolution, literature, and film: A reader*. New York: Columbia University Press, 184–193.

Ealy, G. T. (Spring 1994). Of ear trumpets and a resonance plate: Early hearing aids and Beethoven's hearing perception. *19th-Century Music*, 17(3), 262–273.

Earhart, G. M. (2009). Dance as therapy for individuals with Parkinson disease. *The European Journal of Physical and Rehabilitation Medicine*, 45(2), 231–238.

Ehrenzweig, A. (1971). *The hidden order of art: A study in the psychology of artistic imagination*. Berkeley: University of California Press.

Eliade, M. (1965). *Rites and symbols of initiation: The mysteries of birth and rebirth*. W. R. Trask (trans.). New York: Harper & Row (original work published 1958 as *Birth and Rebirth*).

Eliade, M. (1969a). *Images and symbols: Studies in religious symbolism*. P. Mairet (trans.). New York: Sheed and Ward.

Eliade, M. (1969b). *Patanjali and yoga*. C. L. Markmann (trans.). New York: Shocken Books.

Eliade, M. (1975). *Myths, rites, symbols*, vol. 1. W. C. Beane & W. G. Doty (eds.). New York: Harper & Row.

Eliot, A. (1957). *Three hundred years of American painting*. New York: Time.

Ellamil, M., Dobson, C., Beeman, M. & Christoff, K. (2012). Evaluative and generative modes of thought during the creative process. *NeuroImage*, 59, 1783–1794.

Ellena, E. & Huebner, B. (2009). *I remember better when I paint: Treating Alzheimer's through the creative arts therapies* [DVD]. Montreuil: French Connection Films/Hilgos Foundation.

Ellenberger, H. (1970). *The discovery of the unconscious*. New York: Basic Books.

Ellis, L. B. (1892). *History of New Bedford and its vicinity 1602–1892*. Syracuse: D. Mason.

Emery, N. J. & Clayton, N. S. (2004). The mentality of crows: Convergent evolution of intelligence in corvids and apes. *Science*, 306(5703), 1903–1907.

Emotional Unconscious. (2007). In *APA dictionary of psychology*. https://diction ary.apa.org.

Espinel, C. H. (2007). Memory and the creation of art: The syndrome, as in de Kooning, of "Creating in the midst of dementia": An "ArtScience" study of creation, its "Brain Methods" and results. In J. Bogousslavsky & M. G. Hennerici (eds.), *Neurological Disorders in Famous Artists – Part 2, Frontiers of Neurology and Neuroscience*, 22, 150–168.

Espinel, C. H. (1996). De Kooning's late colours and forms: Dementia, creativity, and the healing power of art. *The Lancet*, 347, 1096–1098.

Fawcett, A. J. & Nicolson, R. I. (1995). Persistent deficits in motor skill of children with dyslexia. *Journal of Motor Behavior*, 27, 235–240.

Feinberg, T. E. & Mallatt, J. (2020). Phenomenal consciousness and emergence: Eliminating the explanatory gap. *Frontiers in Psychology*, 11, 1041.

Feist, G. J. (2010). The function of personality in creativity: The nature and nurture of the creative personality. In J. C. Kaufman & R. J. Sternberg (eds.), *The Cambridge handbook of creativity*. Cambridge: Cambridge University Press, 113–130.

Feldman, J. (2018). *Symbiotic Earth: How Lynn Margulis rocked the boat and started a scientific revolution* [DVD]. Hummingbird Films.

Ferracuti, S., Sacco, R. & Lazzari, R. (1996). Dissociative trance disorder: Clinical and Rorschach findings in ten persons reporting demon possession and treated by exorcism. *Journal of Personality Assessment*, 66(3), 525–539.

Feynman, R. (2001). *"What do you care what other people think?" Further adventures of a curious character*. New York: W. W. Norton.

Finberg, A. J. (1967). *The life of J. M. W. Turner, R. A.* H. F. Finberg (Revision). Oxford: Oxford University Press.

Finke, R. A. (1996). Imagery, creativity, and emergent structure. *Consciousness and Cognition*, 5, 381–393.

Fishburn, F. A., Murty, V. P., Hlutkowsky, C. O. et al. (2018). Putting our heads together: Interpersonal neural synchronization as a biological mechanism for shared intentionality. *Social Cognitive and Affective Neuroscience*, 13(8), 841–849.

Fisher, M. P. A. (2015). Quantum cognition: The possibility of processing with nuclear spins in the brain. *Annals of Physics*, 362, 593–602.

Fisk, J. & Nichols, J. (eds.). (1997). *Composers on music: Eight centuries of writings*, 2nd ed. Boston: Northeastern University Press.

Fitzgerald, P. (2015). *The bookshop*. New York: Mariner Books.

Flam, J. (1986). *Matisse, the man and his art*. Ithaca: Cornell University Press.

Flounders, M. W., González-García, C., Hardstone, R. & He, B. J. (2019). Neural dynamics of visual ambiguity resolution by perceptual prior. *Elife*, 8, e41861.

Foundation for Art and Healing. (2020). https://artandhealing.org.

Fraile, E., Bernon, D., Rouch, I. et al. (2019). The effect of learning an individualized song on autobiographical memory recall in individuals with Alzheimer's disease: A pilot study. *Journal of Clinical & Experimental Neuropsychology*, 41(7), 760–768.

Freud, S. (1963). *The unconscious in general psychological theory: Papers on metapsychology*. New York: Macmillan, 116–150 (original work published 1915).

Freud, S. (1989). *Leonardo da Vinci and a memory of his childhood*. New York: W. W. Norton (original work published 1910).

Froese, T. & Fuchs, T. (2012). The extended body: A case study in the neurophenomenology of social interaction. *Phenomenology and the Cognitive Sciences*, 11, 205–235.

Froese, T., Gershenson, C. & Rosenblueth, D. A. (2013). The dynamically extended mind – A minimal modeling case study. *2013 IEEE Congress on Evolutionary Computation, Cancun, Mexico*, arXiv: 1305.1958,

Futterman Collier, A. & Wayment, H. A. (2021). Enhancing and explaining art-making for mood-repair: The benefits of positive growth-oriented instructions and quiet ego contemplation. *Psychology of Aesthetics, Creativity, and the Arts*, 15(2), 363–376.

Gablik, S. (1970). *Magritte*. Greenwich: New York Graphic Society.

Gabora, L. (2017). Honing theory: A complex systems framework for creativity. *Nonlinear Dynamics, Psychology, and Life Sciences*, 21(1), 35–88.

Gabora, L. & DiPaola, S. (2012). How did humans become so creative? A computational approach. In M. Maher, K. Hammond, A. Pease et al. (eds.), *Proceedings of the Third International Conference on Computational Creativity*. Palo Alto: Association for the Advancement of Artificial Intelligence, 203–210.

Gabora, L. & Kaufman, S. B. (2010). Evolutionary perspectives on creativity. In J. Kaufman & R. Sternberg (eds.), *The Cambridge handbook of creativity*. Cambridge: Cambridge University Press, 279–300.

Gadamer, H.-G. (1977). *Philosophical hermeneutics*. D. E. Linge (trans. & ed.). Berkeley: University of California Press.

Gaev, G. (2021). Licensed social worker. Telephone communication.

Galaburda, A. M. (1983). Developmental dyslexia: Current anatomical research. *Annals of Dyslexia*, 33(1), 41–53.

Galaburda, A. M. (1989). Ordinary and extraordinary brain development: Anatomical variation in developmental dyslexia. *Annals of Dyslexia*, 39, 65–80.

Galanter, P. (2003). What is generative art? Complexity theory as a context for art theory. Presented at GA2003 – 6th Generative Art Conference, Milan, Italy.

Galison, P. L. (1979). Minkowski's space-time: From visual thinking to the absolute world. *Historical Studies in the Physical Sciences*, 10, 85–121.

Garcia-Fenech, G. (2019). Dostoevsky and the challenge of Hans Holbein's Dead Christ. *ARTSTOR*. www.artstor.org.

Gardner, H. (1985). *Frames of mind: The theory of multiple intelligences*. New York: Basic Books.

Garrard, P., Maloney, L. M., Hodges, J. R. & Patterson, K. (2005). The effects of very early Alzheimer's disease on the characteristics of writing by a renowned author. *Brain*, 128(2) 250–260.

Gawley, C. & Palmer, C. (2013). The blindness of others. In C. Palmer (ed.), *The sporting image: Unsung heroes of the Olympics 1896–2012*. Preston: SSTO, 91–94.

Gazzaniga, M. S., Bogen, J. E. & Sperry, R. W. (1962). Some functional effects of sectioning the cerebral commissures in man. *Proceedings of the National Academy of Sciences*, 48(10), 1765–1769.

Gentner, D. (1989). The mechanisms of analogical learning. In S. Vosniadou & A. Ortony (eds.), *Similarity and analogical reasoning*. Cambridge: Cambridge University Press, 199–241.

Ghiselin, B. (ed.). (1985). Introduction. In B. Ghiselin (ed.), *The creative process*. Berkeley: University of California Press, 11–31.

Gibbons, A. (2017). Oldest members of our species discovered in Morocco: New fossils and dates put a face on early Homo sapiens. *Science*, 356(6342), 993–994.

Glisky, M. L., Tataryn, D. J., Tobias, B. A., Kihlstrom, J. F., & McConkey, K. M. (1991). Absorption, openness to experience, and hypnotizability. *Journal of Personality and Social Psychology*, 60(2), 263–272.

Gløersen, I. A. (1994). *Munch as I knew him*. R. Spink (trans.). Hellerup: Edition Bløndal.

Goertzel, B. (1995). Belief systems as attractors. In R. Robertson & A. Combs (eds.), *Chaos theory in psychology and the life sciences*. Mahwah: Erlbaum, 123–134.

Goertzel, V. & Goertzel, M. G. (1962). *Cradles of eminence*. Boston: Little, Brown.

Goldberg, L. R. (1993). The structure of phenotypic personality traits. *American Psychologist*, 48(1), 26–34.

Goleman, D. & Davidson, R. (2017). *Altered traits: Science reveals how meditation changes your mind, brain, and body*. New York: Penguin Random House.

Goodale, M. A. & Milner, A. D. (1992). Separate visual pathways for perception and action. *Trends in Neurosciences*, 15(1), 20–25.

Goodale, M. A. & Westwood, D. A. (2004). An evolving view of duplex vision: Separate but interacting cortical pathways for perception and action. *Current Opinion in Neurobiology*, 14(2), 203–211.

Goodwin, D., Johnston, K., Gustafson, P. et al. (2009). It's okay to be a quad: Wheelchair rugby players sense of community. *Adapted Physical Activity Quarterly*, 26(2), 102–117.

Goodwin, D. L., Krohn, J. & Kuhnle, A. (2004). Beyond the wheelchair: The experience of dance. *Adapted Physical Activity Quarterly*, 21, 229–247.

Goren-Inbar, N. (1986). A figurine from the Acheulean site of Berekhat Ram. *Mitekufat Haeven: Journal of the Israel Prehistoric Society*, 19, 7–12.

Gould, S. J. & Eldredge, N. (Spring 1977). Punctuated equilibria: The tempo and mode of evolution reconsidered. *Paleobiology*, 3(2), 115–151.

Goulden, N., Khusnulina, A., Davis, N. J. et al. (2014). The salience network is responsible for switching between the default mode network and the central executive network: Replication from DCM. *Neuroimage*, 99, 180–190.

Gourfink, M. (2005). This is my house. www.myriam-gourfink.com.

Gowan, J. C. (1975). *Trance, art, and creativity*. Buffalo: Creative Education Foundation.

Grandin, T. (1995). *Thinking in pictures: And other reports from my life with autism*. New York: Doubleday.

Grandin, T. & Johnson, C. (2005). *Animals in translation: Using the mysteries of autism to decode animal behavior*. New York: Scribner.

Gretton, C. & Ffytche, D. H. (2014). Art and the brain: A view from dementia. *International Journal of Geriatric Psychiatry*, 29, 111–126.

Greyson, B. (1997). Near-death narratives. In S. Krippner & S. M. Powers (eds.), *Broken images, broken selves: Dissociative narratives in clinical practice*. Washington: Brunner/Mazel, 163–180.

Griffiths, M. D. (2014). Having an art attack: A brief look at Stendhal syndrome. *Psychology Today*. www.psychologytoday.com.

Grimm, Brothers. (1972). *The complete Grimm's fairy tales*. New York: Pantheon Books (original work published 1812).

Grosso, M. (1997). Inspiration, mediumship, surrealism: The concept of creative dissociation. In S. Krippner & S. M. Powers (eds.), *Broken images, broken selves: Dissociative narratives in clinical practice*. Washington: Brunner/Mazel, 181–198.

Groth, G. (2011). Jack Kirby interview. *The Comics Journal: TCJ Archive*. www .tcj.com.

Gubar, S. (2020). The perseverance of André Watts. *The New York Times*. www .nytimes.com.

Guenther, M. (2017). " . . . The eyes are no longer wild. You have taken the kudu into your mind": The supererogatory aspect of san hunting. *The South African Archaeological Bulletin*, 72(205), 3–16.

Hadoke, T. (2020). David Toole obituary: One of the world's leading disabled dancers with a gift for combining physical power with bewitching delicacy. *The Guardian*. www.theguardian.com.

Hageman, J. J., Peres, J. F. P., Moreira-Almeida, A. et al. (2010). The neurobiology of trance and mediumship in Brazil. In S. Krippner & H. Friedman (eds.), *Mysterious minds: The neurobiology of psychics, mediums and other extraordinary people*. Santa Barbara: Praeger/ABC Clio, 85–111.

Hagerty, M. R., Isaacs, J., Brasington, L. et al. (2013). Case study of ecstatic meditation: fMRI and EEG evidence of self-stimulating a reward system. *Neural Plasticity*, Article ID 653572, 1–12.

Hale, J. R., de Boer, J. Z., Chanton, J. & Spiller, H. A. (2003). Questioning the Delphic Oracle: Overview/An intoxicating tale. *Scientific American*, 289(2), 66–73.

Hallowell, E. M. & Ratey, J. J. (1994). *Driven to distraction*. New York: Pantheon Books.

Hamamoto, M. (2020). Infinite flow dance. www.infiniteflowdance.org.

Hameroff, S. & Penrose, R. (1996). Orchestrated objective reduction of quantum coherence in brain microtubules: The "Orch OR" model for consciousness. In S. R. Hameroff, A. W. Kaszniak & A. C. Scott (eds.), *Toward a science of consciousness – The first Tucson discussions and debates*. Cambridge: MIT Press, 507–540.

Hamilton, E. (1969). *Mythology*. New York: New American Library.

Hamilton, J. (1997). *Turner*. New York: Random House.

Hanh, T. N. (1974). *Zen Keys*. P. Kapleau (trans.). New York: Doubleday

Hardingham-Gill, T. (2021). The man who found the Titanic is on a new quest. *CNN*. www.cnn.com/travel.

Hari, R. & Miiamaaria, V. K. (2009). Brain basis of human social interaction: From concepts to brain imaging. *Physiological Reviews*, 89(2), 453–479.

Harmand, S., Lewis, J. E., Feibel, C. S. et al. (2015). 13.3-million-year-old stone tools from Lomekwi 3, West Turkana, Kenya. *Nature*, 521(7552), 310–315.

Harmon, W. & Rheingold, H. (1984). *Higher creativity: Liberating the unconscious for breakthrough insights*. Los Angeles: Jeremy P. Tarcher.

Harold, E. & Stone, P. (2004). Reverend Gary Davis. *The Association for Cultural Equity*. www.culturalequity.org.

Harris, D. J., Reiter-Palmon, R. & Kaufman, J. C. (2013). The effect of emotional intelligence and task type on malevolent creativity. *Psychology of Aesthetics, Creativity, and the Arts*, 7(3), 237–244.

Harrod, J. B. (2014a). Palaeoart at two million years ago? A review of the evidence. *Arts*, 3, 135–155.

Harrod, J. B. (2014b). MP Gallery – Markings, signs, graphemes. *OriginsNet.org: Researching the Origins of Art, Religion, and Mind*. www.originsnet.org.

Hartt, F. (1987). *History of Italian Renaissance art*. New York: Abrams.

Haseltine, E. (2018). 7 extraordinary feats your brain can perform. *Psychology Today*. www.psychologytoday.com.

Hayes, J. R. (2002). Three problems in teaching general skills. In D. J. Levitan (ed.), *The foundations of cognitive psychology*. Cambridge: MIT Press, 528–541 (original work published 1985).

Heeney, B. (2005). *Bushman shaman: Awakening the spirit through ecstatic dance*. Rochester: Destiny books.

Heidigger, M. (1977). *Basic writings*. D. F. Krell (ed.). New York: Harper & Row.

Heitkamp, H. C., Schmid, K. & Scheib, K. (1993). β-endorphin and adrenocorticotropic hormone production during marathon and incremental exercise. *European Journal of Applied Physiology and Occupational Physiology*, 66, 269–274.

Heneka, M. T., Carson, M. J., El Khoury, J. et al. (2015). Neuroinflammation in Alzheimer's disease. *The Lancet Neurology*, 14(4), 388–405.

Henshilwood, C., d'Errico, F., Vanhaeren, M., van Niekerk, K. & Jacobs, Z. (2004). Middle Stone Age shell beads from South Africa. *Science*, 304(5669), 404–404.

Henshilwood, C. S. (2009). The origins of symbolism, spirituality & shamans: Exploring middle stone age material culture in South Africa. In C. Renfrew & I. Morley (eds.), *Becoming human: Innovation in prehistoric material and spiritual cultures*. Cambridge: Cambridge University Press, 29–49.

Henshilwood, C. S. & d'Errico, F. (2011). Middle Stone Age engravings and their significance to the debate on the emergence of symbolic material culture. In C. S. Henshilwood & F. d'Errico (eds.), *Homo symbolicus: The dawn of language, imagination and spirituality*. Amsterdam: John Benjamins, 75–96.

Henshilwood, C. S., d'Errico, F., van Niekerk, K. L. et al. (2011). A 100,000-year-old ochre-processing workshop at Blombos Cave, South Africa. *Science*, 334 (6053), 219–221.

Henshilwood, C. S., d'Errico, F., van Niekerk, K. L. et al. (2018). An abstract drawing from the 73,000-year-old levels at Blombos Cave, South Africa. *Nature*, 562(7725), 115–118.

Henshilwood, C. S., d'Errico, F. & Watts, I. (2009). Engraved ochres from the Middle Stone Age levels at Blombos Cave, South Africa. *Journal of Human Evolution*, 57(1), 27–47.

Henshilwood, C. S., d'Errico, F., Yates, R. et al. (2002). Emergence of modern human behavior: Middle Stone Age engravings from South Africa. *Science*, 295 (5558), 1278–1280.

Henshilwood, C. & Sealy, J. (1997). Bone artefacts from the middle stone age at Blombos Cave, Southern Cape, South Africa. *Current Anthropology*, 38(5), 890–895.

Henson, R. A. (1988). Maurice Ravel's illness: A tragedy of lost creativity. *British Medical Journal*, 296, 1585–1588.

Heraclitus. (1987). *Fragments: A text and translation*. Commentary by T. M. Robinson. Toronto: University of Toronto Press.

Hesse, J. & Gross, T. (2014). Self-organized criticality as a fundamental property of neural systems. *Frontiers in Systems Neuroscience*, 8, 1–14.

Heyrman, H. (2005). *Art and synesthesia: In search of the synesthetic experience*. Paper presented at the First International Conference on Art and Synesthesia, Universidad de Almería, Spain. www.doctorhugo.org/synaesthesia/art/index .html.

Hickman, R. & Banister, D. (2005). If, at first, the idea is not absurd, then there is no hope for it: Towards 15 MtC in the UK transport sector. Paper presented at the 45th Congress of the European Regional Science Association (ERSA), Amsterdam, The Netherlands. http://hdl.handle.net/10419/117864.

Hirsch, F. & Bell, J. (2014). Birth of the method: The revolution in American acting. *Sight and Sound*, 24(11), 44–51.

Hodgson, D. & Pettitt, P. B. (2018). The origins of iconic depictions: A falsifiable model derived from the visual science of Palaeolithic cave art and world rock art. *Cambridge Archaeological Journal*, 28(4), 591–612.

Holmes, E. (2013). *The life of Mozart.* Kendal: Finkle Street, Kindle ed. (original work published 1845).

Homer, W. I. & Goodrich, L. (1989). *Albert Pinkham Ryder: Painter of dreams.* New York: Harry N. Abrams.

Horden, P. (ed.). (2000). *Music as medicine: The history of music therapy since antiquity.* New York: Routledge.

Houshmand, Z., Harrington, A., Saron, C. & Davidson, R. J. (2002). Training the mind: First steps in a cross-cultural collaboration in neuroscience research. In R. J. Davidson & A. Harrington (eds.), *Visions of compassion: Western scientists and Tibetan Buddhist monks examine human nature.* Oxford: Oxford University Press, 3–17.

Hovers, E. (2009). *The lithic assemblages of Qafzeh Cave.* New York: Oxford University Press.

Hovers, E., Ilani, S., Bar-Yosef, O. & Vandermeersch, B. (2003). An early case of color symbolism: Ochre use by modern humans in Qafzeh Cave. *Current Anthropology*, 44(4), 491–522.

Hovers, E., Vandermeersch, B. & Bar-Yosef, O. (1996). A middle Palaeolithic engraved artefact from Qafzeh Cave, Israel.*Rock Art Research*, 14(2), 79–87.

Huang, J. Y. & Bargh, J. A. (2014). The selfish goal: Autonomously operating motivational structures as the proximate cause of human judgment and behavior.*Behavioral and Brain Sciences*, 37(2), 121–135.

Huber, E., Chang, K., Alvarez, I. et al. (2019). Early blindness shapes cortical representations of auditory frequency within auditory cortex. *Journal of Neuroscience*, 39(26), 5143–5152.

Hultsch, D. F., Hertzog, C., Small, B. J. & Dixon, R. A. (1999). Use it or lose it: Engaged lifestyle as a buffer of cognitive decline in aging? *Psychology and Aging*, 14(2), 245–263.

Hunt, H. T. (1995). *On the nature of consciousness.* New Haven: Yale University Press.

Hupfeld, K. E., Abagis, T. R. & Shah, P. T. (2018). Living "in the zone": Hyperfocus in adult ADHD. *ADHD Attention Deficit and Hyperactivity Disorders*, 11(2), 191–208.

Hutchinson, A. (2018). *Endure: Mind, body and the curiously elastic limits of human performance.* London: HarperCollins.

Huxtable, R. J. (2000). The deafness of Beethoven: A paradigm of hearing problems. *Proceedings of the Western Pharmacology Society*, 43, 1–8.

Huxtable, R. J. (2001). Beethoven: A life of sound and silence. *Molecular Interventions*, 1(1), 8–12.

Inal, S. (2014). Competitive dance for individuals with disabilities. *Palaestra*, 28(1), 31–35.

Isham, H. F. (2004). *Image of the sea: Oceanic consciousness in the romantic century.* Bern: Peter Lang International Academic.

James, W. (1918). *The principles of psychology*, vols. 1 & 2. Gloucester: Pantianos Classics, e-book ed. (original work published 1890).

James, W. (1929). *The varieties of religious experience*. New York: Random House (original work published 1895).

Jamieson, R. W. (1995). Material culture and social death: African American burial practices. *Historical Archaeology*, 29(4), 39–58.

Janouch, G. (2012). *Conversations with Kafka*. G. Rees (trans.). New York: New Directions (original work published 1968).

Jola, C. & Grosbras, M. H. (2013). In the here and now: Enhanced motor corticospinal excitability in novices when watching live compared to video recorded dance. *Cognitive Neuroscience*, 4, 90–98.

Josef, L., Goldstein, P., Mayseless, N., Ayalon, L. & Shamay-Tsoory, S. G. (2019). The oxytocinergic system mediates synchronized interpersonal movement during dance. *Scientific Reports*, 9 (1894), 1–8.

Joufflineau, C., Vincent, C. & Bachrach, A. (2018). Synchronization, attention and transformation: Multidimensional exploration of the aesthetic experience of contemporary dance spectators. *Behavioral Sciences*, 8(2), 24.

Józsa, L. G. (2011). Obesity in the Paleolithic era. *Hormones*, 10(3), 241–244.

Jung, A. (2019). She lifted a car off her dad and saved his life. *Reader's Digest*. www.rd.com.

Jung, C. G. (1963). *Memories, dreams, reflections*. A. Jaffe (ed.), R. Winston & C. Winston (trans.). New York: Random House.

Jung, C. G. (1966). *The spirit in man, art, and literature*. R. F. C. Hull (trans.). Princeton: Princeton University Press, Bollingen Series.

Jung, C. G. (1969). *The archetypes and the collective unconscious*. R. F. C. Hull (trans.). Princeton: Princeton University Press, Bollingen Series.

Jung, C. G. (1971). *On the nature of the psyche*. R. F. C. Hull (trans.). Princeton: Princeton University Press, Bollingen Series.

Jung, C. G. (1972). *Mandala symbolism*. R. F. C. Hull (trans.). Princeton: Princeton University Press, Bollingen Series.

Jung, C. G. (1973). *Four archetypes*. R. F. C. Hull (trans.). Princeton: Princeton University Press, Bollingen Series.

Jung, C. G. (1976). *Symbols of transformation*. R. F. C. Hull (trans.). Princeton: Princeton University Press, Bollingen Series.

Jung, C. G. (1977). *Mysterium coniunctionis*. R. F. C. Hull (trans.). Princeton: Princeton University Press, Bollingen Series.

Jung, C. G. (1978). *Aion: Researches into the phenomenology of the self*. R. F. C. Hull (trans.). Princeton: Princeton University Press, Bollingen Series.

Jung, C. G. (2014). *The collected works of C. G. Jung*. Complete digital edition. H. Read, M. Fordham, G. Adler & W. McGuire (eds.). R. F. C. Hull (trans.). Princeton: Princeton University Press, Bollingen Series.

Kafka, F. (2016). *Letters to friends, family and editors*. R. Winston & C. Winston (trans.). New York: Schocken.

Kaimala, G., Ayaza, H., Herres, J. et al. (2017). Functional near-infrared spectros-copy assessment of reward perception based on visual self-expression: Coloring, doodling, and free drawing. *The Arts in Psychotherapy*, 55, 85–92.

Kallir, O. (1973). *Grandma moses*. New York: Abrams.

Kandinsky, W. (1977). *Concerning the spiritual in art*. M. T. H. Sadler (trans.). New York: Dover (original work published 1914).

Kapchan, D. (2007). *Traveling spirit masters: Moroccan Gnawa trance and music in the global marketplace*. Middletown: Wesleyan University Press.

Kapur, N. (1996). Paradoxical functional facilitation in brain-behaviour research: A critical review. *Brain*, 119(5), 1775–1790.

Kasof, J. (1997). Creativity and breadth of attention. *Creativity Research Journal*, 10 (4), 303–315.

Katz, L. & Berlin, K. S. (2014). Psychological stress in childhood and myopia development. *Optometry & Visual Performance*, 2(6), 289–297.

Kaufman, J. C. & Beghetto, R. A. (2009). Beyond big and little: The four c model of creativity. *Review of General Psychology*, 13(1), 1–12.

Kaufman, S. B. & Gregoire, C. (2016). *Wired to create: Unraveling the mysteries of the creative mind*. New York: Penguin Random House.

Kaufman, S. B., Quilty, L. C., Grazioplene, R. G. et al. (2016). Openness to experience and intellect differentially predict creative achievement in the arts and sciences. *Journal of Personality*, 84(2), 248–258.

Kedar, Y., Kedar, G. & Barkai, R. (2021). Hypoxia in Paleolithic decorated caves: The use of artificial light in deep caves reduces oxygen concentration and induces altered states of consciousness. *Time and Mind: The Journal of Archaeology, Consciousness and Culture*, 14(2), 1–36.

Keele, K. D. (1984). Leonardo da Vinci the anatomist. In *Leonardo da Vinci: Anatomical drawings from the Royal Library Windsor Castle*. Catalog for an exhibition at the Metropolitan Museum of Art. New York: The Metropolitan Museum of Art.

Keller, E. F. (1983). *Feeling for the organism: The life and work of Barbara McClintock*. New York: W. H. Freeman.

Keller, H. (1996). *The story of my life*. Mineola: Penguin; Dover (original work published 1903).

Kellermann, N. P. (2013). Epigenetic transmission of Holocaust trauma: Can nightmares be inherited? *Israel Journal of Psychiatry and Related Sciences*, 50(1), 33–39.

Kent, R. (1939). *World-famous paintings*. New York: Wm. H. Wise.

Khoury & Weltman. (2004). Chameleon cosmology. *Physical Review D (PRD)*. 69, 044026, 1–25.

Kihlstrom, J. F. (1987). The cognitive unconscious. *Science*, 237(4821), 1445–1452.

Kihlstrom, J. F. (2008). The automaticity juggernaut. In J. Baer, J. C. Kaufman & R. F. Baumeister (eds.), *Are we free? Psychology and free will*. New York: Oxford University Press, 155–180.

Killingsworth, M. A. & Gilbert, D. T. (2010). A wandering mind is an unhappy mind. *Science*, 330, 932.

Kilteni, K., Andersson, B. J., Houborg, C. & Ehrsson, H. H. (2018). Motor imagery involves predicting the sensory consequences of the imagined movement. *Nature Communications*, 9(1617), 1–9.

Kirk, A. & Kertesz, A. (1991). On drawing impairment in Alzheimer's disease. *Archives of Neurology*, 48, 73–77.

Klee, P. (1969). *Paul Klee on modern art*. P. Findlay (trans.). London: Faber and Faber (original work published 1948).

Klein, M. (1996). Notes on some schizoid mechanisms. *Journal of Psychotherapy Practice and Research*, 5(2), 163–183 (original work published 1946).

Klein, R. G. (1995). Anatomy, behavior, and modern human origins. *Journal of World Prehistory*, 9(2), 167–201.

Kleisiaris, C. F., Sfakianakis, C. & Papathanasiou, I. V. (2014). Health care practices in ancient Greece: The Hippocratic ideal. *Journal of Medical Ethics and History of Medicine*, 7(6), 1–5. https://pubmed.ncbi.nlm.nih.gov.

Klumpke, A. (1997). *Rosa Bonheur: The artist's (auto)biography*. G. van Slyke (trans.). Ann Arbor: University of Michigan Press.

Kohls, N., Sauer, S., Offenbächer, M. & Giordano, J. (2011). Spirituality: An overlooked predictor of placebo effects? *Philosophical Transactions of the Royal Society B*, 366, 1838–1848.

Kohn, M. & Mithen, S. (1999). Handaxes: Products of sexual selection? *Antiquity*, 73(281), 518–526.

Kontos, P. C. (2003). "The painterly hand": Embodied consciousness and Alzheimer's disease. *Journal of Aging Studies*, 17, 151–170.

Kotler, S. (2014). Flow states and creativity: Can you train people to be more creative? *Psychology Today*. www.psychologytoday.com.

Kounios, J. & Beeman, M. (2015). *The eureka factor: Creative insights and the brain*. London: Windmill Books.

Kounios, J., Fleck, J. I., Green, D. L. et al. (2008). The origins of insight in resting-state brain activity. *Neuropsychologia*, 46(1), 281–291.

Kozbelt, A., Beghetto, R. A. & Runco, M. A. (2019). Theories of creativity. In J. C. Kaufman & R. J. Sternberg (eds.), *The Cambridge handbook of creativity*. Cambridge: Cambridge University Press, 20–47.

Kozicz, M. (2017). Sea shells and tombs: Burial rituals from Senegal to New Orleans. *Via Nola Vie*. www.vianolavie.org.

Krippner, S. (1997a). Dissociation in many times and places. In S. Krippner & S. M. Powers (eds.), *Broken images, broken selves: Dissociative narratives in clinical practice*. Washington: Brunner/Mazel, 3–40.

Krippner, S. (1997b). The varieties of dissociative experiences. In S. Krippner & S. M. Powers (eds.), *Broken images, broken selves: Dissociative narratives in clinical practice*. Washington: Brunner/Mazel, 336–361.

Krippner, S. (1999a). Altered and transitional states. In M. A. Runco & S. R. Pritzger (eds.), *Encyclopedia of creativity*. San Diego: Academic Press, 59–70.

Krippner, S. (1999b). Dreams and creativity. In M. A. Runco & S. R. Pritzger (eds.), *Encyclopedia of creativity*. San Diego: Academic Press, 597–606.

Krippner, S. (1999c). The varieties of dissociative experience: A transpersonal, postmodern model. *The International Journal of Transpersonal Studies*, 18(2), 81–101.

Krippner, S. (2002). Shamanism as a spiritual technology. *Journal of Religion & Psychical Research*, 25(1), 52–58.

Krippner, S. (2005). Trance and the trickster: Hypnosis as a liminal phenomenon. *International Journal of Clinical and Experimental Hypnosis*, 53(2), 97–118.

Krippner, S. (2008). The role played by mandalas in Navajo and Tibetan rituals. *Anthropology of Consciousness*, 8(1), 22–31.

Krippner, S. & Combs, A. (Autumn 2000a). Self-organization in the dreaming brain. *The Journal of Mind and Behavior*, 21(4), 399–412.

Krippner, S. & Combs, A. (2002b). The neurophenomenology of shamanism. *Journal of Consciousness Studies*, 9(3), 77–82.

Kris, E. (1971). *Psychoanalytic explorations in art*. New York: Schocken (original work published 1952).

Kruglanski, A. & Gigerenzer, G. (2011). Intuitive and deliberate judgments are based on common principles. *Psychological Review*, 118(1), 97–109.

Kubba, A. K. & Young, M. (1996). Ludwig van Beethoven: A medical biography. *The Lancet*, 347(8995), 167–170.

Kubota, I. (1984). A personal chronology by Itchiku Kubota. In T. Yamanobe (ed.), *Opulence: The kimonos and robes of Itchiku Kubota*. Tokyo: Kodansha International, 128–130.

Kumpf, T. (1993). One vet to another: Interview with Ernie Pepion. In *Ernie Pepion – Dreams on wheels*. Missoula: Missoula Museum of the Arts.

Lacey, M. (2012). After promoting others' work, a late-blooming sculptor realizes her dream. *The New York Times*. www.nytimes.com.

Langley, M., Clarkson, C. & Ulm, S. (2008). Behavioural complexity in Eurasian Neanderthal populations: A chronological examination of the archaeological evidence. *Cambridge Archaeological Journal*, 18(3), 289–307.

Langton, C. (1992). Life at the edge of chaos. In C. G. Langton, C. Taylor, J. D. Farmer & S. Rasmussen (eds.), *Artificial life II, SFI studies in the sciences of complexity*, vol. 10. Reading: Addison Wesley, 41–91.

Lazar, S. W., Kerr, C. E., Wasserman, R. H. et al. (2005). Meditation experience is associated with increased cortical thickness. *NeuroReport*, 16, 1893–1897.

Leakey, L. S. B., Tobias, P. V. & Napier, J. R. (1964). A new species of the genus homo from Olduvai Gorge. *Nature*, 202, 7–9.

Leonardo da Vinci. (1970a). *The notebooks of Leonardo da Vinci*, vol. 1. J. P. Richter (trans. & ed.). New York: Dover (original work published c. 1489–1519).

Leonardo da Vinci. (1970b). *The notebooks of Leonardo da Vinci*, vol. 2. J. P. Richter (trans. & ed.). New York: Dover (original work published c. 1489–1519).

Leonardo da Vinci. (1983). *Leonardo on the human body*. C. D. O'Malley & J. B. de C. M. Saunders (trans. & intro.). New York: Dover (original work published c. 1489–1519).

Leonardo da Vinci. (1989). *Leonardo on painting*. M. Kemp (ed.), M. Kemp & M. Walker (trans.). New Haven: Yale University Press (original work published c. 1489–1519).

Leonardo da Vinci. (2005). *Leonardo's notebooks*. H. A. Suh (ed.). New York: Black Dog & Leventhal (original work published c. 1489–1519).

Lerner, B. H. (2006). *When illness goes public: Celebrity patients and how we look at medicine*. Baltimore: Johns Hopkins University Press.

Lesniak, K. T. (2006). The effect of intercessory prayer on wound healing in nonhuman primates. *Alternative Therapies in Health and Medicine*, 12(6), 42–48.

Lévi-Strauss, C. (1970). *The raw and the cooked: Introduction to a science of mythology*, vol. 1. J. & D. Weightman (trans.). London: Jonathan Cape (original work published 1964).

Levine, B. & Land, H. M. (2016). A meta-synthesis of qualitative findings about dance/movement therapy for individuals with trauma. *Qualitative Health Research*, 26(3), 330–344.

Lewis-Williams, D. J. & Clottes, J. (1998). The mind in the cave – the cave in the mind: Altered consciousness in the Upper Paleolithic. *Anthropology of Consciousness*, 9, 13–21.

Li, J. (2017). Woman opens dance company where wheelchairs take center stage, inspired by her own paralysis journey. *Inside Edition*. www.insideedition.com.

Libet, B. (1999). Do we have free will? *Journal of Consciousness Studies*, 6(8–9), 47–57.

Libet, B., Gleason, C. A., Wright, E. W. & Pearl, D. K. (1993). Time of conscious intention to act in relation to onset of cerebral activity (readiness-potential). In B. Libet (ed.), *Neurophysiology of consciousness: Contemporary neuroscientists (Selected papers of leaders in brain research)*. Boston: Birkhäuser, 249–268.

Library of Congress. (2020). The national recording registry 2010. www.loc.gov /programs/national-recording-preservation-board.

Lieberman, P. (2007). The evolution of human speech: Its anatomical and neural bases. *Current Anthropology*, 48(1), 39–66.

Limb, C. J. & Braun, A. R. (2008). Neural substrates of spontaneous musical performance: An fMRI study of jazz improvisation. *PLoS ONE*, 3(2), e1679.

Lindell, A. K. (2011). Lateral thinkers are not so laterally minded: Hemispheric asymmetry, interaction, and creativity. *Laterality*, 16(4), 479–498.

Lippard, L. (1993). Dreams on wheels: Ernie Pepion. In *Ernie Pepion – Dreams on wheels*. Missoula: Missoula Museum of the Arts.

Liu, S., Erkkinen, M. G., Healey, M. L. et al. (2015). Brain activity and connectivity during poetry composition: Toward a multidimensional model of the creative process. *Human Brain Mapping*, 36, 3351–3372.

Loewe, M. & Blacker, C. (eds.). (1981). *Oracles and divination*. London: George Allen & Unwin.

Loiotile, R., Lane, C., Omaki, A. & Bedny, M. (2020). Enhanced performance on a sentence comprehension task in congenitally blind adults. *Language, Cognition and Neuroscience*, 35(8), 1010–1023.

Lombard, M., Högberg, A. & Haidle, M. (2019). Cognition: From capuchin rock pounding to Lomekwian flake production. *Cambridge Archaeological Journal*, 29(2), 201–231.

Loo, S. K., Hale, T. S., Macion, J. et al. (2009). Cortical activity patterns in ADHD during arousal, activation and sustained attention. *Neuropsychologia*, 47 (10), 2114–2119.

Lorenz, E. (1972). *Predictability: Does the flap of a butterfly's wings in Brazil set off a tornado in Texas?* Address at the annual meeting of the American Association for the Advancement of Science, Washington.

Luders, E., Clark, K., Narr, K. L. & Toga, A. W. (2011). Enhanced brain connectivity in long-term meditation practitioners. *NeuroImage*, 57, 1308–1316.

Luders, E., Toga, A. W., Lepore, N. & Gaser, C. (2009). The underlying anatomical correlates of long-term meditation: Larger hippocampal and frontal volumes of gray matter. *NeuroImage*, 45, 672–678.

Ludovise, B. (1986). Inner vision guides this blind swimmer: Mission Viejo's Trischa Zorn proves she deserved her college scholarship. *The Los Angeles Times*. www.latimes.com/archives.

Lujano, B. & Schiro, T. (2014). *No arms, no legs, no problem: When life happens, you can wish to die or choose to live.* Write with Grace, Kindle ed.

Lutz, A., Greischar, L. L., Rawlings, N. B., Ricard, M. & Davidson, R. J. (2004). Long-term meditators self-induce high-amplitude gamma synchrony during mental practice. *Proceedings of the National Academy of Sciences of the United States of America*, 101(46), 16369–16373.

Lutz, A., Slagter, H. A., Dunne, J. D. & Davidson, R. J. (2008). Attention regulation and monitoring in meditation. *Trends in Cognitive Science*, 12(4), 163–169.

Lycett, S. J. (2009). Understanding ancient hominin dispersals using artefactual data: A phylogeographic analysis of Acheulean handaxes. *PLoS ONE*, 4(10), e7404.

Mach, E. (1991). *Great contemporary pianists speak for themselves: Two volumes bound as one.* New York: Dover (original work published 1980 and 1988).

Macdonald, G. (1990). Creative chaos: The dynamics of competitive composition. *Simulation & Gaming*, 21(1), 78–82.

Maclean, J. N. (Autumn 2004). Fire and ashes: The last survivor of the Mann Gulch fire. *Montana: The Magazine of Western History*, 54(3), 18–33.

Maclean, N. (2017). *Young men and fire.* Chicago: University of Chicago Press, Kindle ed. (original work published 1992).

Madill, P. V. (1999). Comments on the "science of symptoms" and the experience of stress. *Advances in Mind-Body Medicine*, 15, 68–72.

Maese, R. (2016). For Olympians, seeing (in their minds) is believing (it can happen). *The Washington Post*. www.washingtonpost.com.

Magherini, G. (1989). *La Sindrome di Stendhal.* Firenze: Ponte Alle Grazie.

Maguire, E. A., Gadian, D. G., Johnsrude, I. S. et al. (2000). Navigation-related structural change in the hippocampi of taxi drivers. *Proceedings of the National Academy of Science*, 97(8), 4398–4403.

Mailer, N. (1973). *Marilyn: A biography*. New York: Grosset & Dunlap.

Mallett, R. L. (2000). Weak gravitational field of the electromagnetic radiation in a ring laser. *Physics Letters A*, 269, 214–217.

Mallett, R. L. (2003). The gravitational field of a circulating light beam. *Foundations of Physics*, 33, 1307–1314.

Mallett, R. L. (2006). *Time traveler: A scientist's personal mission to make time travel a reality*. With B. Henderson. New York: Thunder's Mouth Press.

Mandelbrot, B. B. (1983). *The fractal geometry of nature*. San Francisco: W. H. Freeman.

Mann, T. (2016). Teenager finds super strength to lift burning truck off her dad. *Metro*.https://metro.co.uk.

Maran, M. (ed.). (2013). *Why we write*. New York: Penguin Group.

Marano, R. (2020). Leeds dancer who had legs amputated at 18-months-old and performed for Princess Diana honoured with OBE. *The Yorkshire Evening Post*. www.yorkshireeveningpost.co.uk.

Markoff, I. (2016). Introduction to Sufi music and ritual in Turkey. *Review of Middle East Studies*, 29(2), 157–160. (original work published 1995).

Marks-Tarlow, T. (2008). *Psyche's veil: Psychotherapy, fractals, and complexity*. London: Routledge.

Marks-Tarlow, T. (2020). A fractal epistemology for transpersonal psychology. In T. Marks-Tarlow, Y. Shapiro, K. P. Wolf & H. Friedman (eds.), *A fractal epistemology for a scientific psychology: Bridging the personal with the transpersonal*. Newcastle upon Tyne: Cambridge Scholars, 2–32.

Marron, T. R. & Faust, M. (2018). Free association, divergent thinking, and creativity: Cognitive and neural perspectives. In R. E. Jung & O. Vartanian (eds.), *The Cambridge handbook of the neuroscience of creativity*. Cambridge: Cambridge University Press, 261–280.

Marshack, A. (1996). A Middle Paleolithic symbolic composition from the Golan Heights: The earliest known depictive image. *Current Anthropology*, 37(2), 357–365.

Marshack, A. (1997). The Berekhat Ram figurine: A late Acheulian carving from the Middle East. *Antiquity*, 71(272), 327–337.

Martin, T. C. (1992). *The researches and writings of Nikola Tesla*, 2nd ed. New York: Barnes & Noble Books.

Martineau, K. (2020). Q&A: Markus Buehler on setting coronavirus and AI-inspired proteins to music: Translated into sound, SARS-CoV-2 tricks our ear in the same way the virus tricks our cells. *MIT Quest for Intelligence*. http://news.mit.edu.

Maslow, A. H. (1964). *Religions, values, and peak experiences*. London: Penguin Books.

Matloff, G. L. (2016). Can panpsychism become an observational science? *Journal of Consciousness Exploration & Research*, 7(7), 524–543.

Matsuzawa, T. (1994). Field experiments on use of stone tools by chimpanzees in the wild. In R. W. Wrangham, W. C. McGrew, F. B. M. de Waal & P. G. Heltne (eds.), *Chimpanzee cultures*. Cambridge: Harvard University Press, 351–370.

Mattison, R. S. (2003). *Robert Rauschenberg: Breaking boundaries*. New Haven: Yale University Press.

Mayer, K., Wyckoff, S. N. & Strehl, U. (2016). Underarousal in adult ADHD: How are peripheral and cortical arousal related? *Clinical EEG and Neuroscience*, 47(3), 171–179.

Mayseless, N., Eran, A. & Shamay-Tsoory, S. (2015). Generating original ideas: The neural underpinning of originality. *NeuroImage*, 116, 232–239.

McDermott, J. F. (2000). Emily Dickinson's "nervous prostration" and its possible relationship to her work. *The Emily Dickinson Journal*, 9(1), 71–86.

McKee, M. (2015). Dark energy tested on a tabletop. *Quanta Magazine*. www.quantamagazine.org.

McKendry, M. de la F. (1976). Robert Rauschenberg talks to Maxime de la Falaise McKendry. *Interview*, 6(5), 34, 36.

Mcleod, P. (1995). By swimming beyond barriers, Zorn inspires others: Paralympic games: Blind teacher hopes to encourage people to deal more handily with their disabilities. *LA Times*. www.latimes.com.

McWilliams, M. & Wilson, J. (2015). Home range, body condition, and survival of rehabilitated raccoons (procyon lotor) during their first winter. *Journal of Applied Animal Welfare Science*, 18(2), 133–152.

Meijer, D. K. F. & Geesink, H. J. H. (2017). Consciousness in the universe is scale invariant and implies an event horizon of the human brain. *NeuroQuantology*, 15(3), 41–79.

Meir, B. & Rothen, N. (2013). Synaesthesia and memory. In J. Simner & E. M. Hubbard (eds.), *The Oxford handbook of synesthesia*. Oxford: Oxford University Press, 692–706.

Melzack, R. (1999). From the gate to the neuromatrix. *Pain: A Journal for the International Study of Pain*, 82, S121–S126.

Melzack, R. & Wall, P. D. (1965). Pain mechanisms: A new theory. *Science*, 150 (3699), 971–979.

Mercier, J. (1979). *Ethiopian magic scrolls*. New York: George Braziller.

Mercier, J. (1997). *Art that heals: The image as medicine in Ethiopia*. New York: The Museum for African Art.

Merleau-Ponty, M. (1964). *The primacy of perception*. J. Wild (ed.). Chicago: Northwestern University Press.

Merrotsy, P. (2013). A note on big-C creativity and little-c creativity. *Creativity Research Journal*, 25(4), 474–476.

Messinger, L. M. (Fall 1984). Georgia O'Keeffe. *The Metropolitan Museum of Art Bulletin*, 42(2), 3–58.

Meulenberg, F. (1996). de Kooning's dementia. *The Lancet*, 347, 1838.

Meulenberg, F. (1997). The hidden delight of psoriasis. *British Medical Journal*, 315 (20–27), 1709–1711.

M. H. (2019). Immersion therapy. Why do baths incubate ideas? *The Economist, Prospero*. www.economist.com/prospero.

Michelangelo. (1963). *Complete poems and selected letters of Michelangelo.* R. N. Linscott (ed.), C. Gilbert (trans.). Princeton: Princeton University Press (original work written 1496–1563).

Miller, B. L. (2006). Director, Memory and Aging Center, Weil Institute for Neurosciences, University of California San Francisco. Personal conversation.

Miller, B. L., Boone, K., Cummings, J. et al. (1998). Emergence of artistic talent in frontotemporal dementia. *Neurology*, 51, 978–982.

Miller, B. L., Boone, K., Cummings, J. L., Read, S. L. & Mishkin, F. (2000). Functional correlates of musical and visual ability in frontotemporal dementia. *British Journal of Psychiatry*, 176, 458–463.

Miller, B. L. & Hou, C. E. (2004). Portraits of artists emergence of visual creativity in dementia. *Neurological Review*, 61(6), 842–844.

Miller, B. L., Yener, G. & Akdal, G. (2005). Artistic patterns in dementia. *Journal of Neurological Sciences*, 22(3), 245–249.

Mizuguchi, N., Nakata, H., Uchida, Y. & Kanosu, K. (2012). Motor imagery and sport performance. *The Journal of Physical Fitness and Sports Medicine*, 1(1), 103–111.

Moeckel, R. (2012). Chaos in the three-body problem. Presentation, Poincaré 100 Conference, University of Minnesota. www.math.umn.edu/~rmoeckel/presen tations/PoincareTalk.pdf.

Monge, L. & Evans, D. S. (2003). New songs of Blind Lemon Jefferson. *Journal of Texas Music History*, 3(2), 1–21. https://digital.library.txstate.edu.

Montuori, A., Combs, A. & Richards, R. (2004). Creativity, consciousness, and the direction for human development. In D. Loye (ed.), *The great adventure: Toward a fully human theory of evolution*. Albany: State University of New York Press, 197–236.

Moon, B. (ed.). (1991). *An encyclopedia of archetypal symbolism*, vol. 1. The Archive for Research in Archetypal Symbolism. Boston: Shambhala.

Morriss-Kay, G. M. (2010). The evolution of human artistic creativity. *Journal of Anatomy*, 216(2), 158–176.

Moses, G. (1952). *My life's history*. London: Andre Deutsch.

Moss, D. & Lee, Y. J. (Spring 2012). Dean Moss by Young Jean Lee. *Bomb*, 119, 56–63.

Motluk, A. (2005). Senses special: The art of seeing without sight. *New Scientist*. www.newscientist.com.

Mould, R. F. (2016). Thomas Edison (1847–1931): Biography with special reference to X-rays. *Nowotwory Journal of Oncology*, 66(6), 499–507.

Mozart, W. A. (1985). A letter. In B. Ghiselin (ed.), *The creative process*. Berkeley: University of California Press, 34–35 (original work published 1912).

Mulvenna, C. (2007). Synaesthesia, the arts, and creativity: A neurological connection. In J. Bogousslavsky & M. G. Hennerici (eds.), *Neurological disorders in famous artists – Part 2*. Basel: Karger, 206–222.

Mulvenna, C. (2013). Synaesthesia and creativity. In J. Simner & E. M. Hubbard (eds.), *The Oxford handbook of synesthesia*. Oxford: Oxford University Press, 607–630.

Mumon Ekai. (2008). *The gateless gate: All 48 koans by Ekai, called Mumon.* Weare: Waking Lion Press/Boomer Books (original work published 1228).

Murphy, M. (2020). Art Tatum. *Jazz Profiles* from National Public Radio. https://legacy.npr.org.

Murphy, M. & White, R. A. (1995). *In the zone: Transcendent experience in sports.* New York: Penguin.

Murphy, T. (2019). "Solving the hard problem": Consciousness as an intrinsic property of magnetic fields. *Journal of Consciousness Exploration & Research*, 10 (8), 646–659.

National Aeronautics and Space Administration (NASA). (2017). Collapsing star gives birth to a black hole. *Goddard Space Flight Center.* www.nasa.gov.

National Aeronautics and Space Administration (NASA). (2020a). The energy of empty space. *Space math @ NASA. Goddard Space Flight Center.* www.nasa.gov.

National Aeronautics and Space Administration (NASA). (2020b). Voyager record. *Jet Propulsion Laboratory, California Institute of Technology.* https://voyager.jpl.nasa.gov›golden-record

NBC4 News. (2016). Virginia teen girl lifts truck to rescue father. www.nbcwashington.com.

Nelson, K. P. & Hourigan, R. M. (2016). A comparative case study of learning strategies and recommendations of five professional musicians with dyslexia. *Update: Applications of Research in Music Education*, 35(1), 54–65.

Nelson, S. & Polansky, L. (1993). The music of the Voyager interstellar record. *Journal of Applied Communication Research*, 21(4), 358–376.

Nestler, E. J. (2014). Epigenetic mechanisms of depression. *JAMA Psychiatry*, 71 (4), 454–456.

Neumann, E. (1974). *The great mother.* R. Mannheim (trans.). Princeton: Princeton University Press, Bollingen Series.

Newcomb, A. (2012). Superhero woman lifts car off dad. *ABC News.* https://abcnews.go.com.

Nicolis, G. & Prigogine I. (1989). *Exploring complexity.* New York: W. H. Freeman.

Nietzsche, F. (1985). Composition of "Thus spake Zarathustra." In B. Ghiselin (ed.), *The creative process.* Berkeley: University of California Press, 208–211.

Nietzsche, F. (2017). *Ecce Homo: How one becomes what one is* [Kindle HDX version]. www.amazon.com (original work written 1888, published 1911).

Nietzsche, F. (2020). *Ecce Homo: How one becomes what one is.* A. M. Ludovici (trans.). Boston: Digireads.com (original work published 1911).

Nobel Prize. (2021). Barbara McClintock Nobel lecture. *The Nobel Prize in Physiology or Medicine 1983.* www.nobelprize.org.

Nthala, G. M. (2011). The concept of masking as a cultural device for Chewa music and dance performances. *Journal of the Musical Arts in Africa*, 8(1), 49–73.

NYU Langone Health. (2012). NYU School of Medicine Adult ADHD program to host a special screening of *Gigante: A documentary.* www.newswise.com/articles/nyu-school-of-medicine-adult-adhd-program.

Ogungbile, D. O. (1997). Water symbolism in African culture and Afro-Christian churches. *Journal of Religious Thought*, 53/54(2/1), 21–38.

O'Keeffe, G. (1976). *Georgia O'Keeffe*. New York: Viking Press.

Oken, B. S. (2008). Placebo effects: Clinical aspects and neurobiology. *Brain*, 131 (11), 2812–2823.

Olver, I. N. & Dutney, A. (2012). A randomized, blinded study of the impact of intercessory prayer on spiritual well-being in patients with cancer. *Alternative Therapies in Health and Medicine*, 18(5), 18–27.

Orloff, J. (2017). *The empath's survival guide: Life strategies for sensitive people*. Louisville: Sounds True, Kindle ed.

Osaka, N., Minamoto, T., Yaoi, K. et al. (2015). How two brains make one synchronized mind in the inferior frontal cortex: fNIRS-based hyperscanning during cooperative singing. *Frontiers in Psychology*, 6(1811), 1–11.

Overy, K. (2000). Dyslexia, temporal processing and music: The potential of music as an early learning aid for dyslexic children. *Psychology of Music*, 28(2), 218–229.

Overy, K. (2003). Dyslexia and music: From timing deficits to musical intervention. *Annals of the New York Academy of Sciences*, 999, 497–505.

Pace, D. M. (1993). Blind Arthur Blake. *Blues News*. The Kansas City Blues Society. https://blueskc.org.

Pace, D. M. (1996). Blind Boy Fuller. *Blues News*. The Kansas City Blues Society. https://blueskc.org.

Pais, A. (1991). *Niels Bohr's times: In physics, philosophy, and polity*. Oxford: Oxford University Press.

Palacios-Sánchez, L., Botero-Meneses, J. S., Piñeros-Hernández, L. B., Triana-Melo, J. D. P. & Ramírez-Rodríguez, S. (2018). Stendhal syndrome: A clinical and historical overview. *Arquivos de Neuro-Psiquiatria*, 76(2), 120–123.

Paralympics. (2020a). Mehmet Sefa Ozturk, Turkey para dance sport. www.paralympic.org.

Paralympics. (2020b). Para dance news, World para dance sport. www.paralympic.org.

Park, D. C. (1999). Acts of will? *The American Psychologist*, 54(7), 461.

Patanjali. (2011). *The Yoga-Sutra of Patanjali: A new translation with commentary*. C. Hartranft (trans. & com.). Boston: Shambhala, Kindle ed.

Pearce, R. (1912). Chance and the prepared mind. *Science*, 35(912), 941–956.

Penrose, R. & Hameroff, S. (2011). Consciousness in the universe: Neuroscience, quantum space-time geometry and Orch OR theory. *Journal of Cosmology*, 14. www.journalofcosmology.com.

Pepion, E. (1993). *Ernie Pepion – Dreams on wheels*. Artist's statement, interview with T. Kumpf, and essay by L. Lippard. Missoula: Missoula Museum of the Arts.

Pereira, C. (2016). Frequencies of the Buddhist meditative chant – Om Mani Padme Hum. *International Journal of Science and Research*, 5(4): 761–766.

Pert, C. A. (1997). *Molecules of emotion*. New York: Scribner.

Pert, C. A., Ruff, M. R., Weber, R. J. & Herkenham, M. (1985). Neuropeptides and their receptors: A psychosomatic network. *The Journal of Immunology*, 135 (2), 820–828.

Peterson, D. R., Rossing, T. D. & Canfield, G. H. (1994). Acoustics of the hammered dulcimer, its history, and recent developments. *The Journal of the Acoustical Society of America*, 127th Meeting: Acoustical Society of America, 95 (5), 3002.

Pettit, M. (2010a). The problem of raccoon intelligence in behaviourist America. *British Journal for the History of Science*, 43(3), 391–421.

Pettit, M. (2010b). Raccoon intelligence at the borderlands of science: Is it time to bring raccoons back to the psychology laboratory? *American Psychological Association Monitor on Psychology*, 41(10), 26.

Pfeiffer, J. E. (1982). *The creative explosion*. New York: Harper & Row.

Phiri, V. (Winter 2008). Masks and dances, Mwanapwebo and Maliya: A representation of woman at the center of social change in Zambia. *Signs: Journal of Women in Culture & Society*, 33(2), 449–456.

Pincus, D., Cadsky, O., Berardi, V., Asuncion, C. M. & Wann, K. (2019). Fractal self-structure and psychological resilience. *Nonlinear Dynamics, Psychology, and Life Sciences*, 23(1), 52–78.

Pinker, S. (1999). His brain measured up. *The New York Times Archive*. https:// web.archive.org.

Plimpton, G. (ed.). (1988). *Writers at work 08: The Paris Review interviews*. London: Penguin Books.

Plimpton, G. & Crowther, F. H. (1969). E. B. White, The art of the essay, No. 1. *The Paris Review* (48). www.theparisreview.org.

Poincare, H. (2000). Mathematical creation. *Resonance*, 85–94 (original work published 1908).

Polini, P. (2014). William Utermohlen – the late pictures, 1990–2000. www .williamutermohlen.org.

Pollitzer, A. (1988). *A woman on paper: Georgia O'Keeffe*. New York: Simon and Schuster.

Pool-Goudzwaard, A., Groeneveld, W., Coppieters, M. W. & Waterink, W. (2018). Changes in spontaneous overt motor execution immediately after observing others' painful action: Two pilot studies. *Experimental Brain Research*, 236(8), 2333–2345.

Popova, M. (2019). *Figuring*. New York: Pantheon Books.

Possin, K. L. (2010). Visual spatial cognition in neurodegenerative disease. *Neurocase*, 16(6), 466–487.

Potter, P. (2011). From my rotting body, flowers shall grow, and I am in them, and that is eternity – Edvard Munch. *Emerging Infectious Diseases Journal*, 17(3), 573–574.

Pratley, R., Nicklas, B., Rubin, M. et al. (1994). Strength training increases resting metabolic rate and norepinephrine levels in healthy 50- to 65-yr-old men. *Journal of Applied Physiology*, 76(1), 133–137.

Prigogine, I. & Stengers, I. (1984). *Order out of chaos*. Toronto: Bantam Books.

Prosser, J. (2001). The thick-skinned art of John Updike: "From the journal of a leper." *The Yearbook of English Studies, North American Short Stories and Short Fictions*, 31, 182–191.

Proust, M. (2006). *Remembrance of things past*, vol. 1. C. K. S. Moncrieff (trans.). Hertfordshire: Wordsworth Editions (original work published 1913).

Raichle, M. E., MacLeod, A. M., Snyder, A. Z. et al. (2001). A default mode of brain function. *Proceedings of the National Academy of Sciences*, 98(2), 676–682.

Raichle, M. E. & Snyder, A. Z. (2007). A default mode of brain function: A brief history of an evolving idea. *NeuroImage*, 37, 1083–1090.

Rajmohan, V. & Mohandas, E. (2007). Mirror neuron system. *Indian Journal of Psychiatry*, 49(1), 66–69.

Ramachandran, V. S. & Hubbard, E. M. (2005). Hearing colors, tasting shapes. *Scientific American*. www.sciammind.com.

Ramus, F., Pidgeon, E. & Frith, U. (2003). The relationship between motor control and phonology in dyslexic children. *Journal of Child Psychology and Psychiatry*, 44(5), 712–722.

Rao, K. R. (2005). *Consciousness studies: Cross cultural perspectives*. Jefferson: Mc Farland (original work published 2002).

Rawson, M. B. (1982). Louise Baker and the Leonardo syndrome. *Annals of Dyslexia*, 32, 289–304.

Regents of the University of Michigan. (2020). Dyslexia help. *University of Michigan*. http://dyslexiahelp.umich.edu.

Reichard, G. A. (1977). *Navajo medicine man sand paintings*. New York: Dover (original work published 1939 as *Navajo Medicine Man*).

Remnick, N. & Berenstein, E. (2016). At 100, still running for her life. *The New York Times*. www.nytimes.com.

Rendon, J. (2015). *Upside: The new science of post-traumatic growth*. New York: Touchtone.

Ribeiro, E., Neave, N., Nogueiro Morais, R. et al. (2016). Digit ratio (2D:4D), testosterone, cortisol, aggression, personality and hand-grip strength: Evidence for prenatal effects on strength. *Early Human Development*, 100, 21–25.

Ribowsky, M. (2010). *Signed, sealed, and delivered: The soulful journey of Stevie Wonder*. New York: Wiley, Kindle ed.

Ricard, M. (2003). *Monk dancers of Tibet*. C. Hastings (trans.). Boston: Shambhala.

Richards, R. (ed.). (2007). *Everyday creativity and new views of human nature: Psychological, social, and spiritual perspectives*. Washington: American Psychological Association.

Richards, R. (2018). *Everyday creativity and the healthy mind: Dynamic new paths for self and society*. London: Palgrave Macmillan.

Richards, R. & Goslin-Jones, T. (2018). Everyday creativity. In R. Sternberg & J. Kaufman (eds.), *Nature of human creativity*. New York: Cambridge University Press, 224–245.

Ritz, D. & Charles, R. (2009). *Brother Ray: Ray Charles' own story*. Boston: Da Capo Press, Kindle ed.

Ronnberg, A. & Martin, K. (eds.). (2010). *The book of symbols: Reflections on archetypal images*. Cologne: Taschen.

Root-Bernstein, R. & Root-Bernstein, M. (1999). *Sparks of genius: The 12 thinking tools of the world's most creative people*. New York: Houghton Mifflin Harcourt.

Root-Bernstein, R. & Root-Bernstein, M. (2004). Artistic scientists and scientific artists: The link between polymathy and creativity. In R. J. Sternberg, E. L. Grigorenko & J. L. Singer (eds.), *Creativity: From potential to realization*. Washington: American Psychological Association, 127–151.

Rossalbi, A. W. (1975). *Max Ernst*. D. Larkin (ed.). New York: Ballantine Books.

Rothermel, R. C. (1993). Mann Gulch fire: A race that couldn't be won. USDA Forest Service, Intermountain Research Station, Ogden, Utah, General Technical Report INT-299, 10 pp.

Rouw, R. (2013). Synaesthesia, hyperconnectivity and diffusion tensor imaging. In J. Simner & E. M. Hubbard (eds.), *The Oxford handbook of synesthesia*. Oxford: Oxford University Press, 500–518.

Rowden, T. (2012). *The songs of blind folk: African American musicians and the cultures of blindness*. Ann Arbor: University of Michigan Press.

Rubin, H. A. & Shapiro, D. A. (2005). *Murderball*. Hollywood:ThinkFilm and MTV Films.

Rumelhart, D. E., McClelland, J. L. & PDP Research Group. (1987). *Parallel distributed processing, vol. 1: Foundations*. Cambridge: MIT Press.

Sabel, B. A., Wang, J., Cárdenas-Morales, L., Faiq, M. & Heim, C. (2018). Mental stress as consequence and cause of vision loss: the dawn of psychosomatic ophthalmology for preventive and personalized medicine. *Journal of the European Association for Predictive, Preventive and Personalized Medicine*, 9(2), 133–160.

Saccenti, E., Smilde, A. K. & Saris, W. H. M. (2011). Beethoven's deafness and his three styles. *British Medical Journal*, 343(7837), 1298–1300.

Sadler-Smith, E. (2015). Wallas' four-stage model of the creative process: More than meets the eye? *Creativity Research Journal*, 27(4), 342–352.

Şahin, B., Bozkurt, A., Usta, M. B. et al. (2019). Theory of mind: Development, neurobiology, related areas and neurodevelopmental disorders. *Current Approaches in Psychiatry/Psikiyatride Guncel Yaklasimlar*, 11(1), 24–41.

Samaritter, R. (2018). The aesthetic turn in mental health: Reflections on an explorative study into practices in the arts therapies. *Behavioral Sciences*, 8(41), 1–11.

Samuel, W., Masliah, E., Hill, L. R., Butters, N. & Terry, R. (1994). Hippocampal connectivity and Alzheimer's dementia: Effects of synapse loss and tangle frequency in a two-component model. *Neurology*, 44(11), 2081.

Sandblom, P. (1997). *Creativity and disease*. New York: Marion Boyars.

Sartori, G. (1987). Leonardo da Vinci: Omo sanza lettere. A case of surface dyslexia. *Cognitive Neuropsychology*, 4(1), 1–10.

Schmitt, A. & Falkai, P. (2014). Historical aspects of Mozart's mental health and diagnostic insights of ADHD and personality disorders. *European Archives of Psychiatry and Clinical Neuroscience*, 264, 363–365.

Schnitt, D. (1990). Psychological issues in dancers: An overview. *Journal of Physical Education, Recreation, & Dance*, 61(9), 32–34.

Scholem, G. (1969). *On the Kaballah and its symbolism*. R. Manheim (trans.). New York: Schocken Books (original work published 1960).

Scholem, G. (1987). *Kabbalah*. New York: Dorset Press (original work published 1974).

Scholte, T. (2015). Proto-cybernetics in the Stanislavski system of acting: Past foundations, present analyses and future prospects. *Kybernetes*, 44(8/9), 1371–1379.

Schonbrun, Z. (2018). *The performance cortex: How neuroscience is redefining athletic genius*. New York: Penguin Random House.

Schopenhauer, A. (2014). *The basis of morality*. A. B. Bullock (trans.). Chapel Hill: Project Gutenberg, University of North Carolina (original work published 1840).

Schopenhauer, A. (2021). *On noise*. R. Dircks (trans.). New Delhi: Delhi Open Books (original work published 1851).

Schott, G. D. (1999). Mirror writing: Allen's self-observations, Lewis Carroll's "looking-glass" letters, and Leonardo Da Vinci's maps. *The Lancet*, 354(9196), 2158–2161.

Schott, G. D. & Schott, J. M. (2004). Mirror writing, left-handedness, and leftward scripts. *Archives of Neurology*, 61(12), 1849–1851.

Schuldberg, D. (1999). Chaos theory and creativity. In M. A. Runco & S. R. Pritzger (eds.), *Encyclopedia of creativity*. San Diego: Academic Press, 259–272.

Schwartz, S. A. (2010). Nonlocality and exceptional experiences: A study of genius, religious epiphany, and the psychic. *Explore*, 6(4), 227–236.

Schwartz, S. A. (2018). The role of nonlocal consciousness in creativity and social change. *EC Psychology and Psychiatry*, 7(10), 665–678.

Seaberg, M. (2012). Synesthesia: Was Marilyn Monroe a synesthete? *Psychology Today*. www.psychologytoday.com.

Seahawks.com. (2016). Seahawks fan saves her dad from burning building, goes back to check on Russell Wilson "Fathead." www.seahawks.com/news. https://youtu.be/FcKRlCTDrtI.

Seeley, W. W., Brandy, R. M., Crawford, R. K. et al. (2008). Unravelling Boléro: Progressive aphasia, transmodal creativity and the right posterior neocortex. *Brain*, 131(1), 39–49.

Selberg, S. (2017). Rhinestone cowboy: Alzheimer's, celebrity, and the collusions of self. *American Quarterly*, 69(4), 883–901.

Selkoe, D. J. (2002). Alzheimer's disease is a synaptic failure. *Science*, 789, 298.

Sengupta, S. (2019). Becoming Greta: "Invisible girl" to global climate activist, with bumps along the way. *The New York Times*. www.nytimes.com.

Serlin, I. A. (2007). Theory and practices of arts therapies: Whole person integrative approaches to healthcare. In I. A. Serlin, J. Sonke-Henderson, R. Brandman, & J. Graham-Pole (eds.), *Whole person healthcare, vol. 3: The arts & health*. Westport: Praeger, 107–119.

Serlin, I. A. (2010). Working with trauma in Israel. *The California Psychologist*, 2010, 12–15.

Serlin, I. A. (2022). The transcendent moment. American Psychological Association, Division 32, *Society for Humanistic Psychology Newsletter*.

Seshadri, K. G. (2012). Obesity: A Venusian story of Paleolithic proportions. *Indian Journal of Endocrinology and Metabolism*, 16(1), 134–135.

Sevilla, J. (2019). *Whispering the game forth: The semiotics of tracking and hunting*. Project: Human Ecology (Green Psychology). Ashland: Northland (The Environmental) College Nature and Culture Program.

Shamasundar, C. (2008). Relevance of ancient Indian wisdom to modern mental health: A few examples. *Indian Journal of Psychiatry*, 50(2), 138–143.

Shelley, M. W. (1994). *Frankenstein*. New York: Dover (original work published 1831).

Sheridan, D. (2018). Call me Taka. *Net Magazine*. https://netimesmagazine.co.uk.

Shigeru, M., Lesure, C. & Nóbrega, V. A. (2018). Cross-modality information transfer: A hypothesis about the relationship among prehistoric cave paintings, symbolic thinking, and the emergence of language. *Frontiers in Psychology*, 9, 115.

Sickman, L. & Soper, A. (1956). *Art and architecture of China*. New Haven: Yale University Press.

Siegel, B. B. (2009). *101 exercises for the soul: A divine workout plan for body, mind, and spirit*. Novato: New World Library.

Silvey, R. & Mackeith, S. (2018). The paracosm: A special form of fantasy. In D. C. Morrison (ed.), *Organizing early experience: Imagination and cognition in childhood*. Boca Raton: CRC Press, 173–197 (original work published 1999).

Simmonds-Moore, C. (2020). Synesthesia and the perception of unseen realities. *Journal of Humanistic Psychology*, 6(3), 1–21.

Simner, J. & Carmichael, D. A. (2015). Is synaesthesia a dominantly female trait? *Cognitive Neuroscience*, 6(2–3), 68–76.

Simon, M., Lazzouni, L., Campbell, E. et al. (2020). Enhancement of visual biological motion recognition in early-deaf adults: Functional and behavioral correlates. *PLoS ONE*, 15(8), e0236800.

Simone, N. & Cleary, S. (2003). *I put a spell on you: The autobiography of Nina Simone*. Boston: Da Capo Press (original work published 1992).

Siu-Chi Huang. (1968). Chang Tsai's concept of Ch'i. *Philosophy East and West*, University of Hawai'i Press, 18(4), 113–136.

Soderlund, G., Sikstrom, S. & Smart, A. (2007). Listen to the noise: Noise is beneficial for cognitive performance in ADHD. *Journal of Child Psychology and Psychiatry*, 48(8), 840–847.

Sonke, J. (2011). Music and the arts in health: A perspective from the United States. *Music and Arts in Action*, 3(2), 5–14.

Sonnenstrahl, D. M. (2003). *Deaf artists in America: Colonial to contemporary*. San Diego: Dawn Sign Press.

Sowell, T. (2020). *The Einstein syndrome: Bright children who talk late*. New York: Basic Books, Reprint ed.

Spender, S. (1985). The making of a poem. In B. Ghiselin (ed.), *The creative process*. Berkeley: University of California Press, 113–126 (original work published 1946).

Sperry, R. W. (1982). Some effects of disconnecting the cerebral hemispheres. *Science*, 217, 1223–1226.

Stefanatos, G. A. & Wasserstein, J. (2001). Attention deficit/hyperactivity disorder as a right hemisphere syndrome: Selective literature review and detailed neuropsychological case studies. *Annals of the New York Academy of Sciences*, 931, 172–195. .

Sterrett, E. A. (2014). *The science behind emotional intelligence*. Amherst: HRD Press.

Stewart, E. G. (2002). Vignettes: De Kooning's dementia. *American Journal of Alzheimer's Disease and Other Dementias*, 17(5), 313–319.

Stewart, J. S. (2013). Toward a hermeneutics of doodling in the era of Folly. *Word & Image*, 29(4), 409–427.

Storr, R. (1998). *Tony Smith: Architect, painter, sculptor*. New York: The Museum of Modern Art.

Strauss, M., Ulke, C., Paucke, M. et al. (2018). Brain arousal regulation in adults with attention-deficit/hyperactivity disorder (ADHD). *Psychiatry Research*, 261, 102–108.

Strogatz, S. H. (2003). *Sync: How order emerges from chaos in the universe, nature, and daily life*. New York: Hyperion Books.

Subramaniam, K., Kounios, J., Parrish, T. B. & Jung-Beeman, M. A. (2009). Brain mechanism for facilitation of insight by positive affect. *Journal of Cognitive Neuroscience*, 21(3), 415–432.

Susman, R. L. (Summer 1991). Who made the Oldowan Tools? Fossil evidence for tool behavior in Plio-Pleistocene hominids. *Journal of Anthropological Research*, 47(2), 129–151.

Sutton, P. (ed.). (1988). *Dreamings: The art of aboriginal Australia*. New York: The Asia Society Galleries and George Braziller.

Suzuki, S. (1973). *Zen mind, beginners mind*. New York: John Weatherill.

Suzuki, T. (2020). About Takayuki Suzuki. https://taka-swimmer.com

Svansdottir, H. B. & Snaedal, J. (2006). Music therapy in moderate and severe dementia of Alzheimer's type: A case–control study. *International Psychogeriatrics*, International Psychogeriatric Association, 18(4), 613–621.

Sweet, M. (2019). *Some writer! The story of E. B. White*. Boston: HMH Books for Young Readers (original work published 2016).

Sze, M. (ed. & trans.). (1963). *The mustard seed garden manual of painting*. Princeton: Princeton University Press, Bollingen Series (Facsimile of 1887–1888 Shanghai edition of *Chieh Tzu Yuan Hua Chuan*, original work published 1679–1701).

Szymanski, C., Pesquita, A., Brennan, A. A. et al. (2017). Teams on the same wavelength perform better: Inter-brain phase synchronization constitutes a neural substrate for social facilitation. *NeuroImage*, 152, 425–436.

Tang Chün-i. (1956). Chang Tsai's theory of mind and its metaphysical basis. *Philosophy East and West*, University of Hawai'i Press, 6(2), 113–136.

Tangentiality. (2007). In *APA dictionary of psychology*. https://dictionary.apa.org.

Tarr, B., Launay, J. & Dunbar, R. I. M. (2014). Music and social bonding: "Self-other" merging and neurohormonal mechanisms. *Frontiers of Psychology*, 5, 1096. www.frontiersin.org.

Tart, C. T. (ed.). (1990). *Altered states of consciousness.* New York: Harper Collins.

Taylor, R. (2004). Pollock, Mondrian and the nature: Recent scientific investigations. *Chaos Complexity Letters,* 1(3), 265–277.

Taylor, S. (2012). Transformation through suffering: A study of individuals who have experienced positive psychological transformation following periods of intense turmoil. *Journal of Humanistic Psychology,* 52(1), 30–52.

Tchaikovsky, M. I. (1906). *The life & letters of Peter Ilyich Tchaikovsky.* R. Newmarch (ed.). London: John Lane the Bodley Head.

Tedeschi, R. G., Shakespeare-Finch, J., Taku, K. & Calhoun, L. G. (2018). *Posttraumatic growth: Theory, research, and applications.* New York: Routledge.

Tellegen, A. & Atkinson, G. (1974). Openness to absorbing and self-altering experiences ("absorption"), a trait related to hypnotic susceptibility. *Journal of Abnormal Psychology,* 83(3), 268–277.

Texier, P.-J., Porraz, G., Parkington, J. et al. (2010). A Howiesons Poort tradition of engraving ostrich eggshell containers dated to 60,000 years ago at Diepkloof Rock Shelter, South Africa. *Proceedings of the National Academy of Sciences of the United States of America,* 107(14), 6180–6185.

Thomas, R., Sanders, S., Doust, J., Beller, E. & Glasziou, P. (2015). Prevalence of attention-deficit/hyperactivity disorder: A systematic review and meta-analysis. *Pediatrics,* 135(4), 2014–3482.

Thompson, J. J., Ritenbaugh, C. & Nichter, M. (2009). Reconsidering the placebo response from a broad anthropological perspective. *Culture, Medicine & Psychiatry,* 33(1), 112–152.

Thompson, L. J. (1969). Language disabilities in men of eminence. *Bulletin of the Orton Society,* 19, 113–118.

Thunberg, G. (@GretaThunberg). (2019a). Today is #AutismAwarenessDay . Proud to be on the spectrum! [Comment]. *Facebook.* www.facebook.com/gretathunbergsweden/posts/802407010127121.

Thunberg, G. (@GretaThunberg). (2019b). Before I started school striking I had no energy, no friends and I didn't speak to anyone. [Tweet]. *Twitter.* https://twitter.com/GretaThunberg/status/1167916177927991296.

Tierradentro-García, L. O., Botero-Meneses, J. S. & Talero-Gutiérrez, C. (2018). The sound of Jacqueline du Pré: Revisiting her medical and musical history. *Multiple Sclerosis Journal – Experimental, Translational and Clinical,* 4(2).

Tomalin, C. (2012). *Charles Dickens: A life.* New York: Penguin Books (original work published 2011).

Tomasello, M., Kruger, A. C. & Ratner, H. H. (1993). Cultural learning. *Behavioral and Brain Sciences,* 16, 495–552.

Tooby, J. & Cosmides, L. (2005). Evolutionary psychology: Conceptual foundations. In D. M. Buss (ed.), *Handbook of evolutionary psychology.* New York: Wiley, 5–67.

Tooby, J. & Cosmides, L. (2010). Does beauty build adapted minds? Toward an evolutionary theory of aesthetics, fiction, and the arts. In B. Boyd, J. Carroll & J. Gottshall (eds.), *Evolution, literature, and film: A reader.* New York: Columbia University Press, 174–183.

Trance. (2007). In *APA dictionary of psychology*. https://dictionary.apa.org.

Travis, F. & Shear, J. (2010). Focused attention, open monitoring and automatic self-transcending: Categories to organize meditations from Vedic, Buddhist and Chinese traditions. *Consciousness & Cognition*, 19(4), 1110–1118.

Travis, F. & Wallace, R. K. (1999). Autonomic and EEG patterns during eyes-closed rest and transcendental meditation practice. *Consciousness and Cognition*, 8(3), 302–318.

Tucker, J. (2001). *Scourge: The once and future threat of smallpox*. New York: Atlantic Monthly Press.

Tutter, A. (ed.). (2017). *The muse: Psychoanalytic explorations of creative inspiration*. New York: Routledge.

Tymoszuk, U., Perkins, R., Fancourt, D. & Williamon, A. (2019). Cross-sectional and longitudinal associations between receptive arts engagement and loneliness among older adults. *Social Psychiatry and Epidemiology*, 55(7), 891–900.

Tzelepis, A., Schubiner, H. & Warbasse, L. H. (1995). Differential diagnosis and psychiatric comorbidity patterns in adult attention deficit disorder. In K. G. Nadeau (ed.), *A comprehensive guide to attention deficit disorder in adults: Research, diagnosis, treatment*. New York: Brunner/Mazel, 37–39.

Uffizi Galleries. (2020). *The baptism of Christ* by Andrea del Verrocchio. www.uffizi.it/en.

Uleman, J. (2005). Becoming aware of the new unconscious. In R. R. Hassin, J. S. Uleman & J. A. Bargh (eds.), *The new unconscious*. New York: Oxford University Press, 3–15.

Unconscious. (2007). In *APA dictionary of psychology*. https://dictionary.apa.org.

University College London (UCL). (2017). Audience members' hearts beat together at the theatre. *UCL Psychology and Language Sciences*. www.ucl.ac.uk.

University of Massachusetts Amherst (UMass Amherst). (2011). Obituary: Richard Yarde, Art professor, acclaimed watercolorist. *Office of News & Media Relations/ UMass Amherst*. www.umass.edu.

Updike, J. (1996). *The centaur*. New York: Random House (original work published, 1962).

Utermohlen, P. (2006). Details. *William Utermohlen*. www.williamutermohlen.org.

Valencia, A. L. & Froese, T. (2020). What binds us? Inter-brain neural synchronization and its implications for theories of human consciousness. *Neuroscience of consciousness*, 2020(1), 1–12, niaa010.

Valladas, H., Clottes, J., Geneste, J.-M. et al. (2001). Evolution of prehistoric cave art. *Nature*, 413(6855), 479.

Van Campen, C. (2010). *The hidden sense: Synesthesia in art and science*. Cambridge: MIT Press, Leonardo Reprint ed.

Van Campen, C. (2013). Synesthesia in the visual arts. In J. Simner & E. M. Hubbard (eds.), *The Oxford handbook of synesthesia*. Oxford: Oxford University Press, 631–646.

Vandermeersch, B. (2002). The excavation of Qafzeh. *Bulletin du Centre de recherche français à Jérusalem*, 10, 65–70.

Vandewalle, G., Collignon, O., Hull, J. T. et al. (2013). Blue light stimulates cognitive brain activity in visually blind individuals. *Journal of Cognitive Neuroscience*, 25(12), 2072–2085.

van Duijl, M., Kleijn, W. & de Jong, J. (2013). Are symptoms of spirit possessed patients covered by the DSM-IV or DSM-5 criteria for possession trance disorder? A mixed-method explorative study in Uganda. *Social Psychiatry & Psychiatric Epidemiology*, 48, 417–430.

van Duijl, M., Kleijn, W. & de Jong, J. (2014). Unravelling the spirits' message: A study of help-seeking steps and explanatory models among patients suffering from spirit possession in Uganda. *International Journal of Mental Health Systems*, 8(1), 1–13.

Vanhaeren, M., d'Errico, F., Stringer, C. et al. 2006). Middle Paleolithic shell beads in Israel and Algeria. *Science*, 312(5781), 1785–1788.

Van Wittenberghe, I. C. & Peterson, D. C. (2020). Neuroanatomy, corticospinal tract lesion. In *StatPearls* [Internet]. Treasure Island: StatPearls. www.ncbi.nlm.nih.gov.

Varela, F., Lachaux, J. P., Rodriguez, E. & Martinerie, J. (2001). The brainweb: Phase synchronization and large-scale integration. *Nature Reviews Neuroscience*, 2, 229–239.

Vartanian, O. (2009). Variable attention facilitates creative problem solving. *Psychology of Aesthetics, Creativity, and the Arts*, 3(1), 57–59.

Vartanian, O. (2018). Openness to experience: Insights from personality neuroscience. In R. E. Jung & O. Vartanian (eds.), *The Cambridge handbook of the neuroscience of creativity*. Cambridge: Cambridge University Press, 464–475.

Vasari, G. (1996). *The lives of the artists*, vol. 1. G. Du C. De Vere (trans.). New York: Alfred A. Knopf (original work published 1568).

Vecce, C. (2003). Word and image in Leonardo's writing. In C. C. Bambach (ed.), *Leonardo da Vinci: Master draftsman*, The Metropolitan Museum of Art. New Haven: Yale University Press, 59–77.

Vermeij, G. (1977). The Mesozoic marine revolution: Evidence from snails, predators and grazers. *Paleobiology*, 3(3), 245–258.

Vermeij, G. (1994). The evolutionary interaction among species: Selection, escalation, and coevolution. *Annual Review of Ecology and Systematics*, 25(1), 219–236.

Vermeij, G. (1997). *Privileged hands: A scientific life*. New York: W. H. Freeman.

Vernon, M. (2019). Divine transports: Whether via music, dance or prayer, the trance state was key to human evolution, forging society around the transcendent. M. Benjamin (ed.). *Aeon*. https://aeon.co/essays.

Volkow, N. & Swanson, J. M. (2013). Adult attention deficit-hyperactivity disorder. *New England Journal of Medicine*, 369(20), 1935–1944.

Von Franz, M.-L. (1978). *Creation myths*. Zurich: Spring.

Vorwerg, L. (2019). Rehearsing interdisciplinarity: Training, production, practice and the 10,000 hour problem. In M. Evans, K. Thomaidis & L. Worth (eds.), *Time and performer training*. Philadelphia: Taylor & Francis, e-book.

Voss, P., Lassonde, M., Gougoux, F. et al. (2004). Early- and late-onset blind individuals show supra-normal auditory abilities in far-space. *Current Biology*, 14(19), 1734–1738.

Wagner, R. (2004a). *My life*, vol. 1. Chapel Hill: The Project Gutenberg EBook.

Wagner, R. (2004b). *My life*, vol. 2. Chapel Hill: The Project Gutenberg EBook.

Waldrop, M. M. (1992). *Complexity: The emerging science at the edge of order and chaos*. New York: Simon & Shuster.

Wallas, G. (1926). *The art of thought*. London: Jonathan Cape.

Wan, C. Y., Wood, A. G., Reutens, D. C. & Wilson, S. J. (2010). Early but not late-blindness leads to enhanced auditory perception. *Neuropsychologia*, 48(1), 344–348.

Wasserstein, J., Wolf, L. E., Solanto, M., Marks, D. & Simkowitz, P. (2008). Adult attention deficit hyperactivity disorder: Basic and clinical issues. In J. E. Morgan & J. H. Ricker (eds.), *Studies on neuropsychology, neurology and cognition: Textbook of clinical neuropsychology*. London: Psychology Press, 679–695.

Watkins, J. G. & Watkins, H. H. (1997). *Ego states: Theory and therapy*. New York: Norton.

Wegner, D. M. (2005). Who is the controller of controlled processes? In R. R. Hassin, J. S. Uleman & J. A. Bargh (eds.), *The new unconscious*. New York: Oxford University Press, 19–36.

Wegner, D. M. & Wheatley, T. (1999). Apparent mental causation: Sources of the experience of will. *American Psychologist*, 54(7), 480–492.

Weinstein, G. (2017). *Einstein's pathway to the special theory of relativity*, 2nd ed. Newcastle upon Tyne: Cambridge Scholars.

West, T. G. (1992). A future of reversals: Dyslexic talents in a world of computer visualization. *Annals of Dyslexia*, 42(1), 124–139.

West, T. G. (1997). *In the mind's eye: Visual thinkers, gifted people with Dyslexia and other learning difficulties, computer images and the ironies of creativity*. Amherst: Prometheus Books.

White, H. A. & Shah, P. (2006). Uninhibited imaginations: Creativity in adults with attention-deficit/hyperactivity disorder. *Personality and Individual Differences*, 40(6), 1121–1131.

White, R. A. (1997). Dissociation, narratives, and exceptional human experiences. In S. Krippner & S. M. Powers (eds.), *Broken images, broken selves: Dissociative narratives in clinical practice*. Washington: Brunner/Mazel, 88–121.

Whitman, R. D., Holcomb, E. & Zanes, J. (2010). Hemispheric collaboration in creative subjects: Cross-hemisphere priming in a lexical decision task. *Creativity Research Journal*, 22(2), 109–118.

Widiger, T. A. & Costa, P. T. (2012). Integrating normal and abnormal personality structure: The five-factor model. *Journal of Personality*, 80(6), 1471–1505.

Winkelman, M. (2002). Shamanism and cognitive evolution (with comments). *Cambridge Archaeological Journal*, 12(1), 71–101.

Winkelman, M. (2011). Shamanism and the evolutionary origins of spirituality and healing. *NeuroQuantology*, 9(1), 54–71.

Winterson, J. (1997). *Art objects: Essays on ecstasy and effrontery.* New York: Vintage.

Wise, J. (2009a). *Extreme fear: The science of your mind in danger.* New York: Palgrave Macmillan.

Wise, J. (2009b). When fear makes us superhuman. *Scientific American.* www.scientificamerican.com.

Wolfradt, U. & Pretz, J. (2001). Individual differences in creativity: Personality, story writing, and hobbies. *European Journal of Personality*, 15, 297–310.

Wolfram, S. (1984). Computer software in Science and Mathematics. *Scientific American*, 9(84), 188–203.

Woolaver, L. (1995). *The illuminated life of Maud Lewis.* Photographs by Bob Brooks. Halifax: Nimbus/The Art Gallery of Nova Scotia.

Woolaver, L. (1997). *Christmas with Maud Lewis.* Photographs by Bob Brooks. Fredericton: Goose Lane Editions.

Worcester Art Museum. (2003a). Richard Yarde: Ringshout. Past exhibitions. www.worcesterart.org/exhibitions.

Worcester Art Museum. (2003b). Worcester Art Museum exhibition features new work by Richard Yarde. Press release. www.worcesterart.org/news.

Wordsworth, W. (1985). Preface to the second edition of lyrical ballads. In B. Ghiselin (ed.), *The creative process.* Berkeley: University of California Press, 81–82 (original work published 1895).

World Health Organization (WHO). (1992). *ICD-10: The ICD-10 classification of mental and behavioural disorders: Clinical descriptions and diagnostic guidelines.* Geneva: World Health Organization.

World Health Organization (WHO). (2019). Dementia. www.who.int.

World Health Organization (WHO). (2020). Deafness and hearing loss. *World Health Organization Newsroom.* www.who.int/news-room.

Wright, D. J., McCormick, S. A., Birks, S., Loporto, M. & Holmes, P. S. (2015). Action observation and imagery training improve the ease with which athletes can generate imagery. *Journal of Applied Sport Psychology*, 27(2), 156–170.

Wright, P. A. (1997). History of dissociation in western psychology. In S. Krippner & S. M. Powers (eds.), *Broken images, broken selves: Dissociative narratives in clinical practice.* Washington: Brunner/Mazel, 41–60.

Yadon, C. A., Bugg, J. M., Kisley, M. A. & Davalos, D. B. (2009). P50 sensory gating is related to performance on select tasks of cognitive inhibition. *Cognitive, Affective & Behavioral Neuroscience*, 9(4), 448–458.

Yamakoshi, G. & Sugiyama, Y. (1995). Pestle-pounding behavior of wild chimpanzees at Bossou, Guinea: A newly observed tool using behavior. *Primates*, 36 (4), 489–500.

Yarde, R. (2006). Personal communication, telephone interview.

Yehuda, R., Daskalakis, N. P., Lehrner, A. et al. (2014). Influences of maternal and paternal PTSD on epigenetic regulation of the glucocorticoid receptor gene in holocaust survivor offspring. *American Journal of Psychiatry*, 171(8), 872–880.

Zabelina, D. L., O'Leary, D., Pornpattananangkul, N., Nusslock, R. & Beeman, M. (2015). Creativity and sensory gating indexed by the P50:

Selective versus leaky sensory gating in divergent thinkers and creative achievers. *Neuropsychologia*, 69(77), 77–84.

Zatorrea, R. J. & Salimpoora, V. N. (2013). From perception to pleasure: Music and its neural substrates. *Proceedings of the National Academy of Sciences of the United States of America*, 110(supplement), 10430–10437.

Zausner, T. (1996). The creative chaos: Speculations on the connection between nonlinear dynamics and the creative process. In W. Sulis & A. Combs (eds.), *Nonlinear dynamics in human behavior: Studies of nonlinear phenomena in life science*, vol. 5. Singapore: World Scientific, 343–349.

Zausner, T. (1999). Trembling and transcendence: Chaos theory, panic attacks, and awe. *Psychotherapy Patient*, 11 (1–2), 83–107 and In E. M. Stern & R. B. Marchesani (eds.), *Awe and trembling: Psychotherapy of unusual states*. Binghamton: Haworth Press, 83–107.

Zausner, T. (2007). Artist and audience: Everyday creativity and visual art. In R. Richards (ed.), *Everyday creativity and new views of human nature: Psychological, social, and spiritual perspectives*. Washington: American Psychological Association, 75–89.

Zausner, T. (2011a). Chaos, creativity, and substance abuse: The nonlinear dynamics of choice. *Nonlinear Dynamics, Psychology, and Life Sciences*, (15)2, 207–227.

Zausner, T. (2011b). Transcending the self through art: Altered states of consciousness and anomalous events during the creative process. *Journal of Consciousness Exploration & Research*, 2(7), 889–1022.

Zausner, T. (2011–2012). Creativity, resilience, and chaos theory. *DTAA Dance Therapy Association of Australia Journal, Moving On*, 10(1&2), 39–41.

Zausner, T. (2016). *When walls become doorways: Creativity and the transforming illness*, new edition as e-book (Kindle DX version). www.amazon.com (original hardcover ed. 2006).

Zausner, T. (2022). Embracing the infinite: Creativity and the nonlinear self. In D. Schuldberg, R. Richards & S. Guisinger (eds.), *Nonlinear psychology: Keys to chaos and creativity in mind and life*. Oxford: Oxford University Press, 215–226.

Zetlin, M. (2018). In a single sentence of her google doodle, Dr. Jane Goodall teaches a life lesson we all need to learn. www.inc.com.

Zion, S. R. & Crum, A. J. (2018). Mindsets matter: A new framework for harnessing the placebo effect in modern medicine. In L. Colloca (ed.), *International review of neurobiology*. Cambridge: Academic Press, 137–160.

Index

For EU product safety concerns, contact us at Calle de José Abascal, 56–1°,
28003 Madrid, Spain or eugpsr@cambridge.org.

www.ingramcontent.com/pod-product-compliance
Ingram Content Group UK Ltd.
Pitfield, Milton Keynes, MK11 3LW, UK
UKHW020306140625

459647UK00006B/67